Bringing Pain Relief to Children

Bringing Pain Relief to Children

Treatment Approaches

Edited by

G. Allen Finley, MD, FRCPC, FAAP

Departments of Anesthesia and Psychology
Dalhousie University and IWK Health Centre
Halifax, Nova Scotia, Canada

Patrick J. McGrath, OC, PhD, FRSC

Departments of Psychology, Pediatrics, and Psychiatry
Dalhousie University and IWK Health Centre
Halifax, Nova Scotia, Canada

and

Christine T. Chambers, PhD

Departments of Pediatrics and Psychology
Dalhousie University and IWK Health Centre
Halifax, Nova Scotia, Canada

HUMANA PRESS ✳ TOTOWA, NEW JERSEY

© 2006 Humana Press Inc.
999 Riverview Drive, Suite 208
Totowa, New Jersey 07512
www.humanapress.com

Due diligence has been taken by the publishers, editors, and authors of this book to assure the accuracy of the information published and to describe generally accepted practices. The contributors herein have carefully checked to ensure that the drug selections and dosages set forth in this text are accurate and in accord with the standards accepted at the time of publication. Notwithstanding, as new research, changes in government regulations, and knowledge from clinical experience relating to drug therapy and drug reactions constantly occurs, the reader is advised to check the product information provided by the manufacturer of each drug for any change in dosages or for additional warnings and contraindications. This is of utmost importance when the recommended drug herein is a new or infrequently used drug. It is the responsibility of the treating physician to determine dosages and treatment strategies for individual patients. Further it is the responsibility of the health care provider to ascertain the Food and Drug Administration status of each drug or device used in their clinical practice. The publisher, editors, and authors are not responsible for errors or omissions or for any consequences from the application of the information presented in this book and make no warranty, express or implied, with respect to the contents in this publication.

This publication is printed on acid-free paper. ∞

ANSI Z39.48-1984 (American Standards Institute) Permanence of Paper for Printed Library Materials.

Cover Illustration: Getty Images.

Cover design by Patricia F. Cleary

Production Editor: Amy Thau

For additional copies, pricing for bulk purchases, and/or information about other Humana titles, contact Humana at the above address or at any of the following numbers: Tel.: 973-256-1699; Fax: 973-256-8314; E-mail: orders@humanapr.com, or visit our Website: http://www.humanapress.com

Printed in the United States of America. 10 9 8 7 6 5 4 3 2 1
eISBN: 1-59745-125-8
Library of Congress Cataloging in Publication Data
Bringing pain relief to children : treatment approaches / edited by G.
   Allen Finley, Patrick J. McGrath, and Christine T. Chambers.
      p. ; cm.
   Includes bibliographical references and index.
   ISBN 1-58829-628-8 (alk. paper)
   1. Pain in infants--Treatment. 2. Pain in children--Treatment.
   3. Pain in adolescence--Treatment.   I. Finley, G. Allen, 1954-   .
   II. McGrath, Patrick J. III. Chambers, Christine T.
   [DNLM: 1. Pain--therapy--Adolescent. 2. Pain--therapy--Child.
   3. Pain--therapy--Infant. 4. Adolescent Health Services. 5. Child
   Health Services.   WL 704 B858 2006]
   RJ365.B75 2006
   618.92'0472--dc22
                                                                                    2005029432

Preface

Since the 1970s, when the classic study by Eland *(1)* illustrated the significant discrepancy in how pain in children was managed as compared with adults, issues related to the delivery of pain care to children have been at the forefront of research and practice. It is now clear that treatment is possible in most cases of pediatric pain. Although much remains to be done to improve the science of pain relief, the bigger challenge is using science to bring pain relief to all children who are in need.

Some aspects of delivering pain relief to children have received scant attention. Although the location of most studies on pain relief can be found or inferred in the literature, there has generally been little attention to place in pediatric pain research. The setting in which pain is detected and managed is of major importance. For example, pain that is encountered in a tertiary, palliative care setting is both quantitatively and qualitatively different from the pain encountered in the primary care physician's office. Moreover, the skills of the health care providers, the resources, and the therapeutic opportunities differ markedly across different settings. Consider for a moment the resources available in a regional clinic in a developing country and the resources available at one of the quaternary care facilities in North America or Europe. Although it is unlikely that the pharmacokinetics of morphine would differ by place, most other aspects of pain management are likely to be impacted. Understanding the role of place in pain assessment and management is imperative; *Bringing Pain Relief to Children: Treatment Approaches* puts pediatric pain in its place.

Historically, pain management was delivered in medical settings by the physician and medical team assigned to the child. Over the last decade, however, specialized teams and other treatment resources for pain care have emerged. Chapters 1 through 3 (by Drs. McClain, Schechter, and Collins and Frager) of *Bringing Pain Relief to Children: Treatment Approaches* explore the modern-day versions of more traditional hospital-based pain management, including inpatient, outpatient, and palliative care.

In addition, as the impact of children's pain on all facets and quality of life has been better understood, the importance of extending the provision of pain services to children to other environments has been recognized. Chapters 4 and 5 (by Drs. Eccleston et al. and Brown) discuss school and residential settings and the opportunities they provide for the delivery of pain care.

Increasingly, we need to challenge our more traditional approaches to pain management by considering alternate approaches and removing barriers to care. New approaches to treatment have arisen outside of the medical setting.

Chapter 6 (by Dr. Tsao et al.) describes how complementary and alternative medicine approaches can be used to improve pain care. In Chapter 7, McGrath and colleagues detail the as-yet-unfulfilled promise of technology in bringing pain relief to children and youth.

Research on pediatric pain care has almost exclusively focused on children and adolescents in the developed world. However, most children live in the developing world, and it is likely that the risk and prevalence of pain is greater there. Moreover, the current opportunities for treatment are few. Chapter 8 (Finley and Forgeron) tackles this nascent area of research and practice.

In Chapter 9, Drs. Scott-Findlay and Estabrooks bring a much-needed focus on the theory and explicit practice of knowledge dissemination. This understanding is critical regardless of the setting in which pain management is being delivered.

These chapters were derived from the keynote talks given at the Fifth International Forum on Pediatric Pain at White Point Beach in Nova Scotia, Canada, in fall 2004. We were delighted with the vigorous interplay of ideas that occurred during this meeting. The chapters reflect this knowledge exchange.

The children of the world deserve better pain treatment than they currently receive. We hope *Bringing Pain Relief to Children: Treatment Approaches* will help you bring pain relief to all children.

G. Allen Finley, MD, FRCPC, FAAP
Patrick J. McGrath, OC, PhD, FRSC
Christine T. Chambers, PhD

REFERENCE

1. Eland JM, Anderson JE. The experience of pain in children. In: Jacox AK, ed., Pain: A Source Book for Nurses and Other Health Professionals. Boston: Little, Brown, 1977, pp. 453–473.

Acknowledgments

We thank McNeil Consumer Products Canada who supported the Fifth International Forum on Pediatric Pain with an unrestricted educational grant, and Kelly Hayton for her assistance in preparing this book.

Contents

ix

Contributors

RONALD T. BROWN, PhD, ABPP • *Departments of Public Health, Psychology, and Pediatrics, Temple University, Philadelphia, PA*

NICOLA CARMICHAEL, MA (Cantab) • *The Royal National Hospital for Rheumatic Diseases NHS Foundation Trust, Bath, United Kingdom*

CHRISTINE T. CHAMBERS, PhD • *Departments of Pediatrics and Psychology, Dalhousie University and IWK Health Centre, Halifax, Nova Scotia, Canada*

JOHN J. COLLINS, MBBS, PhD, FAChPM, FRACP • *Pain and Palliative Care Service, Children's Hospital at Westmead, Sydney, New South Wales, Australia*

HANNAH CONNELL, D. ClinPsych • *Pain Management Unit, University of Bath and The Royal National Hospital for Rheumatic Diseases NHS Foundation Trust, Bath, United Kingdom*

CHRISTOPHER ECCLESTON, PhD • *Pain Management Unit, University of Bath and The Royal National Hospital for Rheumatic Diseases NHS Foundation Trust, Bath, United Kingdom*

CAROLE A. ESTABROOKS, RN, PhD • *Faculty of Nursing, University of Alberta, Edmonton, Alberta, Canada*

G. ALLEN FINLEY, MD, FRCPC, FAAP • *Departments of Anesthesia and Psychology, Dalhousie University and IWK Health Centre, Halifax, Nova Scotia, Canada*

PAULA A. FORGERON, RN, MN • *Pediatric Pain Management, IWK Health Centre and School of Nursing, Dalhousie University, Halifax, Nova Scotia, Canada*

GERRI FRAGER, MD, FRCPC • *Department of Pediatrics, Dalhousie University and Pediatric Palliative Care, IWK Health Centre, Halifax, Nova Scotia, Canada*

BRENDA C. MCCLAIN, MD, FAAP • *Departments of Anesthesiology and Pediatrics, Yale University School of Medicine, New Haven, CT*

PATRICK J. MCGRATH, OC, PhD, FRSC • *Departments of Psychology, Pediatrics and Psychiatry, Dalhousie University and IWK Health Centre, Halifax, Nova Scotia, Canada*

MARCIA MELDRUM, PhD • *John C. Liebeskind History of Pain Collection, Louise M. Darling Biomedical Library, University of California, Los Angeles, Los Angeles, CA*

ERIN MOON, BA • *Department of Psychology, Dalhousie University and Pain Research Lab, IWK Health Centre, Halifax, Nova Scotia, Canada*

NEIL L. SCHECHTER, MD • *Pain Relief Program, Connecticut Children's Medical Center and Department of Pediatrics, University of Connecticut School of Medicine, Hartford, CT*

SHANNON SCOTT-FINDLAY, RN, MN, PhD (c) • *Faculty of Nursing, University of Alberta, Edmonton, Alberta, Canada*

JENNIE C. I. TSAO, PhD • *Pediatric Pain Program, Department of Pediatrics, David Geffen School of Medicine at University of California, Los Angeles, Los Angeles, CA*

CAROLYN WATTERS, PhD • *Faculty of Computer Science and Graduate Studies, Dalhousie University, Halifax, Nova Scotia, Canada*

LONNIE K. ZELTZER, MD • *Pediatric Pain Program, Departments of Pediatrics, Anesthesiology, Psychiatry, and Biobehavioral Sciences, David Geffen School of Medicine at University of California, Los Angeles, Los Angeles, CA*

1

Hospital-Based Pain Care for Infants and Children

Brenda C. McClain

Summary

Some view acute, in-hospital pain management as within the purview of a said specialty. However, hospital-based pain care for children is more than associated symptom management of a given disease. This chapter demonstrates the complexity of pediatric in-hospital pain management and indicates acute pain syndromes as major components of the specialty of pain medicine. The practice of hospital-based pediatric pain care requires a vast knowledge base that also encompasses the philosophies and skills of chronic pain medicine. The essentials of neurobiology, pharmacology, and practice principles of hospital-based pain care for children are the focus of this chapter.

Key Words: Acute pain; hospital-based pain care; neurobiology; pain management; pediatric.

The aim of this chapter is to present the complexity of hospital-based pain concerns for children. The fund of knowledge required to manage the spectrum of pain that one encounters in hospital-based care supports the need to recognize acute pain as an integral component of the specialty of pain medicine. Currently, certification in pain management and pain medicine requires in-depth knowledge in chronic pain syndromes and cancer-related pain experiences *(1)*. In-hospital acute pain management is often equated to management of perioperative and trauma-related pain and is seen as having a narrow scope of practice and a limited period of patient interaction. According to the European chapter of the International Association for the Study of Pain (IASP), acute pain is relegated to symptom management of a given disease and thus is within the purview of said specialty *(2)*. In addition, the demarcation between the pediatric acute and chronic pain experience is often dismissed in the adult literature, in which medical textbooks relegate the topic to a single chapter on pediatric pain. An understanding

From: *Bringing Pain Relief to Children: Treatment Approaches*
Edited by: G. A. Finley, P. J. McGrath, and C. T. Chambers © Humana Press Inc., Totowa, NJ

of pain neurobiology, pharmacology, and practice principles as they pertain to pediatrics is required.

Training in pain medicine as a specialty should include education and exposure to acute, in-hospital pain syndromes as an essential component of the learning process. Acute pain service personnel must have a broad knowledge base and skill set to handle the in-hospital pain experience. The acute pain service concept has been skewed to represent merely manning watch over epidural and patient-controlled anesthesia (PCA) regimens, as evidenced by reviews of the adult literature on the efficacy of pain services *(3)*. Hospital-based pain management would be better described as the specialty of hospital-based *pain medicine* because care goes beyond techniques. The argument has been made for the application of a multidisciplinary approach in acute pain management *(4)*.

For the purpose of this chapter, the term *hospital-based pain care* is defined as the management of types of pain commonly encountered during hospitalization. Thus, infants and children admitted to the hospital with acute, recurrent, or chronic pain undergo pain intervention through the clinical application of recognized pain management principles.

The utility and efficacy of organized acute pain services have been questioned in the adult arena. The merits of organized pediatric pain services have not been delineated. The impression that hospital-based pain is acute, is limited to the hospitalization period, and thus has a known end point is not always true. Many children and families may be in the hospital for weeks or even months with no clear end in sight *(5–8)*. Children with sudden onset of disease may have a prolonged disease course with associated pain caused by the disease, procedures, and or therapies. Many children who die in the hospital are more likely to have prolonged hospitalizations *(8)*.

Complex hospital-based pediatric pain management is seen in the care of patients with systemic lupus erythematosus, familial pancreatitis, toxic megacolon, scleroderma, and sickle cell disease, to name a few disease processes *(9–12)*. These diseases can seem resistant to standard therapy or have contraindications for high-dose opioid therapy, yet exacerbations of pain may be the primary reason for hospital admissions.

1. The Pediatric Pain Experience

The magnitude of the problem of inadequate pain treatment in children was brought to light in the late 1980s when studies in various institutions independently confirmed that children were undertreated despite the caregivers' recognition of the presence of pain *(13,14)*. The incidence of pediatric pain is unknown because most studies addressed either one specific type of pain or pain treatment and not the general presence and intensity of pain. Anxiety during blood sampling via venipuncture has been cited as a major cause of distress for children. Up to

64% of children 3–6 years old expressed distress about blood sampling; 52% of children 7–17 years old expressed pain *(15)*. Shapiro studied 454 medical-surgical adult inpatients and found that 79% reported experiencing pain during hospitalization *(16)*. A similar study by Donovan and coworkers found that more than half considered their pain excruciating *(17)*. It is reasonable to assume a similar experience in the medical-surgical pediatric population.

Long-term adverse effects have been noted in children who experience greater severity of illness or invasive procedures. A prospective cohort study of 120 pediatric intensive care unit and medical–surgical ward patients revealed that 17.5% of all hospitalized patients expressed significant medical fears 6 weeks postdischarge, and 14% continued to demonstrate clinically significant fear at 6 months postdischarge. The younger the child was, the greater the likelihood of emotional trauma was, as demonstrated by the development of intrusive thoughts and avoidance behaviors *(18)*. Children in the intensive care setting had limited recall of severe pain; children on general wards who had undergone procedure-related pain expressed hesitation and dread of future painful events *(18)*. Prompt and effective analgesic administration attenuates the occurrence of posttraumatic stress disorder in burn-related trauma *(19)*.

Pain intervention is required from humane and scientific points of view. Current literature supports the likelihood of long-term detrimental effects of poorly treated acute pain. Neuroplasticity expressed as central sensitization and hyperalgesia may result from repeated and unopposed noxious stimuli *(20)*. Whether this facilitation of nociception persists indefinitely is unclear, and further longitudinal studies are in order. The full implications of inadequate pain control are unknown. Taddio and colleagues showed that preemptive analgesia before a noxious stimulus can decrease distress in future experiences. Their landmark study revealed that infants who underwent penile block before circumcision experienced limited distress in subsequent vaccinations months later when compared with infants who did not receive preemptive anesthetic blockade before circumcision *(21)*.

The use of nonpharmacological techniques (e.g., distraction) and pharmacological agents must take into consideration the neurobiology of pain and the impact of age and past painful experiences on present response.

2. The Ontogeny of Pain Neurobiology

The development of nociceptive pathways, receptors, and receptor ligands has been best studied in animal models. The observed response to pain in the neonate is variable and is caused by multiple issues in brain development and gestational age at birth. Preterm neonates at 29 and 35 weeks gestational age have a less-robust response to noxious stimuli than do full-term infants *(22)*. There is little human data on the topic, and research has relied mainly on animal models, with the staged development of the rat pup as the accepted model. A rat pup at P7 (day 7 of life) is comparable to a full-term infant and at P21 is comparable to a human adult *(23,24)*. Conflicting research on the induction of endogenous opioid system activity from nutritive and nonnutritive suckling exists. Early studies suggested that orogustatory response to sucrose water caused release of endogenous opioids. Recent studies found no change in measured opioid ligand concentrations after suckling. Furthermore, the ontogeny of opioid receptors and their ligands is not uniform. μ and κ receptors appear much earlier than δ receptors, and the endogenous opioid ligands (endorphins, enkephalins, and dynorphins) appear before receptors are present *(25)*. In addition, in the rat pup descending inhibitory pathways are present at birth but are not functional before day 10 of life *(23)*. Thus, extrapolating from the animal model, the human preterm or even full-term neonate may have a heightened physiochemical response to noxious stimuli because the existing endogenous opioids appear to be incapable of participating in descending inhibitory modulation to diminish the pain response *(25)*.

3. Pain Physiology

Pain is a multifaceted occurrence of sensory, emotional, behavioral, and autonomic responses to actual or potential tissue damage *(26)*. Physiologically, noxious stimuli cause release of biochemical substances that activate free nerve endings called nociceptors. Nociceptive pathways are intact by the second trimester. Incomplete myelination only implies slower conduction. Thus, most preterm infants have the capacity for pain activity *(27)*.

4. The Peripheral System
4.1. Peripheral Nociceptors

The pain receptors are either A-δ or C fibers (Table 1). The A-δ fibers respond to heat and mechanical stress, and the C fibers are polymodal and respond to chemical, mechanical and thermal stimulation. These are further classified as low-threshold mechanoreceptors, high-threshold mechanoreceptors, and high-threshold mechanothermal nociceptors *(28)*.

4.1.1. Deep Somatic and Visceral Nociceptors

The fascia between muscle fibers, tendons, muscles, and their blood vessels are all supplied by A-δ and C fibers. Deep diffuse pain is primarily caused by activation of C fibers. Low- and high-threshold mechanoreceptors are found at articular surfaces. The periosteum of bone is richly innervated. Nociceptors accompany blood vessels in the Haversian canals. Cancellous bone also receives nociceptors *(29)*.

Table 1
Neuronal Fibers and Propagation

Fiber	Innervation	Mean diameter (μm)	Mean conduction velocity (m/s)
Aα	Primary muscle spindle motor to skeletal muscle	15	100
Aβ	Cutaneous touch and pressure	8	50
Aγ	Motor to muscle spindle	6	20
Aδ	Mechanoreceptors, nociceptors, thermoreceptors	3	15
B	Sympathetic preganglionic	3	7
C	Mechanoreceptors, nociceptors, thermoreceptors; sympathetic postganglionic	1	1

Adapted from ref. *150.*

Table 2
Opioid Conversion

Drug	Intravenous (mg)	By mouth (mg)
Morphine (Roxanol, MSIR)	10	30
Hydromorphone (Dilaudid)	1.5	7.5
Oxycodone (Percocet)	15	30
Hydrocodone (Vicodin)	—	30
Levorphanol (Levo-Dromoran)	2	4
Oxymorphone (Numorphan)	1	10
Meperidine (Demerol)	75	—
Fentanyl (Sublimaze)	0.1	—
Methadone (Dolophine)	10	20

Adapted from refs. *151* and *152.*

Visceral pain is not evoked by all viscera, it is not linked to visceral injury, it may be referred, it is diffuse and poorly localized, and it is accompanied by motor and autonomic reflexes *(30)* (Table 2). Dizziness, orthostasis, diaphoresis, and nausea can accompany paroxysmal pain. Therefore, visceral pain can be associated with symptoms of impending doom because of the autonomic symptoms *(31)*.

5. The Central System

5.1. The Dorsal Horn

Dorsal horn neurons can be divided into three types: projecting neurons that transfer sensory information, propriospinal neurons that transfer intersegmental spinal cord input, and local interneurons that are predominantly inhibitory. These inhibitory interneurons contain γ-aminobutyric acid (GABA) and glycine. The main transmitter between peripheral afferents and the dorsal horn is α-amino-3-hydroxyl-5-methyl-4-isoxazole proprionic acid. Subunits of the α-amino-3-hydroxyl-5-methyl-4-isoxazole proprionic acid receptor have been shown to play a role in central sensitization and decreased pain thresholds *(32)*.

5.1.1. The Endogenous Opiate System

There are three classes of opioids: enkephalins, dynorphins, and the β-endorphins. In the rat pup model, opioid ligands appear before opioid receptors are established. The ontogeny of the endogenous opioid system suggests that neonates may have a variable response to painful stimuli caused by immaturity of the endogenous opioid system *(25)*.

Inadequate pain intervention in early life may have long-lasting effects that can persist into adulthood. The immature sensory system of the neonate has a lower threshold for excitation, decreased ability for modulation at the dorsal horn, and plasticity of peripheral and central sensory neuronal structures. The hyperexcitable state may not be clinically apparent in the extremely premature infant. The vigor of the response is partly dependent on vagal tone *(22,32–34)*.

6. Physicochemical Basis of Pain Intervention

Pain management can be approached by intervening at various points of the nociceptive pathway. *Transduction* is the conversion of the peripheral stimulus at the nociceptor into an electrical signal *(35)*. Agents that have been shown to work at the periphery include nonsteroidal anti-inflammatory agents and capsaicin. *Transmission* is the afferent ascendance of the electrical signal from the periphery to the neuraxis. Local anesthetics temporarily block transmission. *Modulation* (i.e., inhibition or facilitation) occurs at the level of the interneurons and supraspinal pathways *(36)*. Opioids, tricyclic antidepressants (TCAs), and GABA agonists are some of the agents effective in manipulating suppression of perceived pain *(37)*.

7. Pharmacological Concerns

7.1. Drug Distribution

The total drug concentration is composed of free un-ionized drug fraction and the protein-bound ionized fraction. The degree of ionization is dynamic and is dependent on the pH of the environment and whether the drug is a weak acid or weak base. The aqueous form is necessary to gain access to the lipid membrane; the un-ionized form crosses the lipid membrane. Drugs bind to specific and nonspecific plasma proteins. Only free drug is available to interact with active sites *(38)*.

Albumin is a protein receptor with a large capacity but low affinity for most drugs. α-1-Acid glycoprotein has a low capacity but high affinity for binding drugs. Fentanyl binds α-1-acid glycoprotein. The concentration of α-1-acid glycoprotein is affected by age and disease *(39)*. Variable concentration of this protein is usually of little consequence except in the neonate because they have low levels of α-1-acid glycoprotein.

7.1.1. Drug Absorption

Enteric (e.g., orogastric and rectal) uptake of drugs is by passive diffusion and bulk flow. Liquid preparations will have a more rapid rate of absorption than tablets or capsules, but the speed of diffusion is not affected by form. The rate of diffusion is determined by the amount of surface area available, the pH of gastric fluid, and the rate of gastric emptying. The rate of gastric emptying can be affected by the presence of surgical conditions, drugs, and food. Once transit to the small intestine occurs, the drug is available for absorption for 6 hours *(40)*. Rectal suppositories have an erratic uptake that is partly dependent on the level of placement. The superior rectal vein in the upper region is connected to the portal system, and drugs placed high above the dentate line undergo hepatic first pass. The lower region of the rectum is supplied by the inferior and middle rectal veins, which directly connect to the systemic circulation *(41)*.

The intravenous route is the most direct and avoids the barriers of hepatic first-pass metabolism and tissue absorption. However, some drugs cause pain on intravascular injection. The discomfort can be lessened by slowing the rate of injection or by dilution of the drug in volume or with simultaneous infusion of maintenance fluids. Analgesics known to cause discomfort on injection, especially when minimally diluted, include morphine and ketorolac. Sedatives that cause discomfort on injection include diazepam and propofol. Intramuscular injections are discouraged in children because of the anxiety and pain caused by hypodermic injection.

Maintaining peripheral intravenous access can be difficult in neonates and young children because of movement and ease of dislodging relatively small-gage intravenous catheters *(42)*. The oral route should not be forgotten if inadvertent intravenous catheter dislodgement occurs and oral administration is not contraindicated.

8. Philosophy of Pain Intervention

The principles of good pain management are emphasized by the Agency for Health Care Policy and Research guidelines for acute pain management. Despite the availability of both effective pain assessment tools and strategies for minimizing pain, suboptimal pain management and unrelieved pain commonly occur among surgical and medical patients *(43)*.

8.1. Principles of Pediatric Pain Management

Tenets of good pain management for children are as follows: First, give medications by the clock. Around-the-clock administration ensures consistent plasma levels. As-needed (prn, *pro re nata*) administration has been interpreted by staff to mean as little as possible. Suboptimal dosing by 25% as-needed scheduling has been documented in adults *(44)*.

Second, give by the oral route when possible. Novel routes to consider are sublingual, rectal, intranasal, inhalational, and subcutaneous administration. Patients with moderate-to-severe pain often require intravenous delivery of opioids and adjuvants. However, in the presence of emesis or poor intravenous access, novel routes should be considered. Intramuscular administration is less acceptable because fear of needles may result in avoidance of needed analgesia *(45)*.

Third, give analgesics by pain intensity. Mild-to-moderate pain should be managed with nonsteroidal anti-inflammatory drugs (NSAIDs) and oral "weak" opioids. Severe pain is managed by oral "strong" opioids or intravenous opioids and regional blockade techniques. Transdermal systems of opioids have little application in acute pain but are continued if the patient with chronic pain receiving this technique is admitted for acute exacerbation of pain.

Fourth, pain management should consider the patient. Drug choice and administration should be tailored to the patient's age, health, and activity. For example, in the neonate, the physiological and behavioral responses are sensitive indicators of pain, but they have poor specificity. Therefore, pain assessment is affected by the sleep–wake cycle, disease-related stress, or apprehension. When the assessment is equivocal in determining the presence of pain in the neonate, it is better to assume that pain is present and to treat accordingly. Preemptive administration of analgesics is appropriate before the onset of known painful procedure *(46)*. Older infants metabolize and eliminate opioids similar to adults. Continuous infusions of opioids are safe in infants older than 6 months. Plasma levels of morphine remain consistent with stable dosing even when the infusion is continued for several days *(47)*. The use of multimodal techniques and agents potentially decreases the side effects of higher doses of a single-agent technique *(48)*. NSAIDs and α-2 agonists have opioid-sparing effects by reducing the amount of narcotic required and the occurrence of dose-dependent side effects *(49)*. Neuropathic pain is less responsive to opioids and may respond better to membrane-stabilizing agents, such as TCAs and antiepileptic drugs (AEDs). A combination of two or more agents may be required to address various types of pain that contribute to the painful episode.

Finally, one should promptly treat side effects. Opioids form the cornerstone of care for moderate-to-severe pain in all age groups, and adequate knowledge of the pharmacology of individual agents is needed. Side effects of nausea and pruritus are common and should be anticipated and addressed throughout the care plan. Stool stimulants are to be considered when extended use of an opioid is projected. Stool softeners may be inadequate because they do not cause propulsion of feces. Stool stimulants are warranted when defecation is absent after 3 days of opioid administration because tolerance of side effects, such as constipation, can take 1 week or more to occur *(50)*.

8.1.1. Maximizing Benefits Despite Side Effects

Most opioid side effects result from μ receptor activity and should be treated with mu antagonists. Side effects are dose dependent and often respond to a reduction in dose, but this response is slow. The mechanism for pruritus is likely not caused by histamine release, although antihistamines are commonly given. Low-dose naloxone or nalbuphine is used in an around-the-clock or as-needed basis for nausea and pruritus *(51)*.

Sedation and respiratory depression in chronic opioid use can be addressed by rearrangement of dosing schedules or by the addition of psychostimulants such as dextroamphetamine. The nonamphetamine stimulant modafinil, 2-[(diphenylmethyl) sulfanyl] acetamide, has demonstrated efficacy in pediatric cases of daytime sleepiness and narcolepsy and may be beneficial to those patients displaying excessive opioid sedation in the face of good pain control *(52,53)*. Adjuvants, such as TCAs, are added to improve sleep and enhance analgesia.

9. Types of Pain in Hospital-Based Pain Care

The 1992 IASP Task Force on Acute Pain cited the following forms of acute pain as major health concerns: postoperative pain; trauma and burn pain; acutely painful medical conditions (e.g., sickle crisis pain, acute abdominal pain, acute myofascial pain); and acute cancer pain *(54)*. In pediatrics, procedure-related pain is a major component of the cancer pain-related experience.

9.1. Perioperative Pain

Perioperative pain management should address the preoperative, intraoperative, and postoperative phases for comprehensive intervention and the best attempt to limit the unpleasantness of the surgical pain experience. The management of postoperative pain begins in the preoperative period. The degree of postoperative pain is somewhat influenced by the level of preoperative anticipatory distress *(55)*. Open discussion of expectations of the family and child for the postoperative period should be encouraged. Preoperative visits allow the family and child to meet the anesthesiologist, preview the perioperative care suite, and address anxiety concerning anesthesia and surgery. Child life specialists may conduct tours of the recovery and operative areas. Child life specialists also perform medical role play using dolls, puppets, and games. Thus, the use of child life specialists provides a nonthreatening avenue for patient self-expression *(56)*.

Preoperative preparation helps both the child and the family deal with illness, injury, and treatment.

The concept of wind-up was initially presented by Crile and Katz in 1993. The noxious act of surgery causes injury to C fibers and a heightened response to subsequent stimuli and occurs secondary to central sensitization at the wide dynamic-range neurons of Rexed lamina V *(57)*. McQuay performed a systematic review of the literature and found that intrathecal opioid and epidural local anesthetics administered prior to incision decrease pain scores and need for intravenous opioid for the initial 6 hours postoperatively *(58)*. The evidence to date suggests that wound infiltration before surgical incision does not produce preemptive analgesia in muscle-splitting procedures *(59)*.

Theoretically, preemptive prophylactic intervention should attenuate the occurrence of the wind-up phenomenon. There is conflicting data regarding the efficacy of any one drug class or route of analgesic delivery. The existence of wind-up in the pediatric population has been challenged; thus, the efficacy of preemptive analgesia in children has been questioned *(60)*.

NSAIDs may contribute to preemptive analgesia at two locales. NSAIDs act peripherally as anti-inflammatory agents and may possess a central effect on spinal activity mediated by N-methyl-D-aspartate *(61)*. Timing appears important to the efficacy of preemptive analgesia. Intravenous ketoprofen given 30 minutes prior to incision was effective for breast surgery and reduced opioid consumption by more than 40% for up to10 hours in the immediate postoperative period *(61)*.

Oral premedicants given in the immediate preoperative period have decreased postoperative analgesic requirements. Oral clonidine at 5 µg/kg has the ability to lower Visual Analog Scale (VAS) scores and intravenous morphine consumption for orthopedic procedures significantly *(62)*. Oral clonidine was effective in lowering VAS and opioid requirements in abdominal procedures for which postoperative pain was managed by neuraxial analgesia but not by parenteral opioids *(63)*. Midazolam, a water-soluble imidazo-benzodiazepine, has no analgesic properties. Yet, when given preoperatively as a sedative, midazolam causes a decrease in postoperative anxiety and analgesic requirements *(64)*.

Intraoperative pain management most often involves general anesthesia and intravenous opioids. Pediatric regional techniques are often performed after the induction of general anesthesia, in contradistinction to awake techniques in adults. Utilization of regional techniques as the primary anesthetic has been reported by Puncuh et al. *(65)*. Children 6 months to 14 years underwent neuraxial anesthesia; however, sedation was required. General anesthesia may cause postoperative apnea in neonates and infants who have preexisting central or peripheral tendencies for apnea. In these cases, local anesthetics with or without epinephrine are used for intrathecal anesthesia in an attempt to avoid respiratory embarrassment.

Adequate pain control in the immediate postoperative period should be obtained as swiftly as possible to decrease postoperative anxiety. Consistent and repeated pain assessment and intervention must be performed in a timely fashion to ensure effective pain relief. Pain assessment should take into account the degree of pain at rest (static pain) and on activity (dynamic pain) to address the changeable aspects of the pain experience.

Breakthrough pain was first defined in 1989 by Portenoy and Hagen in the analysis of cancer pain *(66)*. Today, this term is also applied in cases of nonmalignant pain *(67)*. The IASP defines *breakthrough pain* as intermittent exacerbations of pain that can occur spontaneously or in relation to specific activity and pain that increases above the level of pain addressed by the ongoing analgesic; the definition includes incident pain and end-of-dose failure *(68)*. Analgesic boluses can be given a few minutes prior to planned activities in an attempt to lessen incident pain. Breakthrough analgesic doses should be titrated independently from the baseline analgesic. Breakthrough pain must be treated with as-needed doses of analgesics in addition to the usual schedule of administration.

9.1.1. Trauma and Burn-Related Pain

According to a US study, the overall incidence of injuries for children 0–19 years old is 2239 per 10,000. The incidence of injuries from burns is relatively low but of greater severity *(69)*. Approximately 40,000 children are hospitalized annually secondary to burn injuries in the United States. Satisfactory pain relief for these children must be considered while other resuscitative measures are undertaken. A survey by Martinez-Herz et al. of 79 burn centers in North America found that analgesics were used less often for control of pain induced by wound care in pediatric patients than adult cases. Of responders, 17% did not use narcotic analgesia in children, and 8% did not recommend analgesia in any form *(70)*.

Judicious administration of opioids is indicated because oversedation may result when standard dosing is used in the face of a reduced volume of distribution. Initially, release of catecholamines after burn injury preserves the blood pressure and heart rate despite the decrease in cardiac output. Subsequently, massive fluid shifts caused by the loss of endothelial integrity result in significant hypovolemia and hemoconcentration. The decline in cardiac output is secondary to the fluid shifts and reduction in venous return. Further decrease in cardiac output occurs despite adequate fluid resuscitation; the decreased output is a result of direct myocardial depression from interleukins, tumor necrosis factor, and oxygen-free radicals *(71)*.

By classification, full-thickness burns involve the destruction of nerve endings at the site of the injury and result in lack of sensation. Contiguous areas are sensitized and painful. Concurrently, in the region of full-thickness burn, some nerve endings are spared, and pain can still be generated *(72)*. Other pain generators include nerve regeneration with associated paresthesia and neuroma formation and nerve entrapment by scar or contractures. The phenomenon of hyperalgesia associated with partial full-thickness thermal injury is characterized by a decrease in the pain threshold and the development of spontaneous pain. This is likely to be mediated by increased sensitization of the A-δ fiber afferents at the site of burn injury *(73)*.

After the burn insult, the activated nerve terminals release the neuropeptides substance P and calcitonin gene-related peptide, which results in vasodilatation. Injured cells also release inflammatory mediators that cause nociceptor activation, which subsequently causes peripheral sensitization in the immediate region of injury (primary hyperalgesia) *(74)*.

There are two types of acute burn-related pain. *Procedural pain* is associated with events involving wound care, such as dressing changes and whirlpool baths. *Background pain* refers to the unpleasant sensation occurring at rest. Underestimation of this latter type of pain could cause the child to suffer more from anxiety and may increase pain intensity experienced during subsequent procedures *(75)*.

Regular assessment of pain is key to managing burn pain. Most burn centers in North America use methods like behavioral observation, monitoring of physical parameters, and parental reports to measure the level of pain. VAS and verbal assessment provide easy grading of pain severity *(76)*. The child's perceptions, level of cognition, and coping behaviors should be regularly assessed and addressed during this period. Accurate measurement of their discomfort is imperative for the development of a proper strategic treatment plan *(77)*.

Aggressive pain management with opioids has been shown to attenuate the development of posttraumatic stress disorder *(19)*. However, analgesic requirements may change after the first 24 hours of burn care because of decreased protein levels and increased bioavailability of free drugs. Because of the shifts in drug availability and physiological instability, administration of opioids requires close observation and frequent pain assessment *(77)*. The treatment plan should address background pain and provide additional dosing for the intense, brief pain associated with procedures. A comprehensive long-term plan for possible chronic pain should be developed before discharge from the hospital.

9.1.1.1. ACUTE MEDICAL PAIN

Many children who require hospital admission first present to the emergency department. The administration of opioid analgesics in patients with acute abdominal pain is frequently limited because of fear of masking symptoms. A survey of 700 board certified or board-eligible pediatric surgeons and emergency medicine physicians revealed that surgeons with more than 10 years of experience were less likely to give analgesics than emergency medicine physicians of comparable experience. The rationale for administering analgesics was based on the literature by 3% of surgeons and 23% of emergency physicians. The majority of emergency physicians who withheld analgesics (64 of 74) stated that disapproval by the surgeon was their main reason for withholding analgesia *(78)*. The use of sonography and computed tomography scan can speed diagnosis such that pain intervention can be readily given without fear of masking symptoms. The many causes of acute abdominal pain are beyond the scope of this chapter. Opioids should be used with caution, however, because diagnostic radiology is not universally utilized, and current evidence is limited.

Johnston et al. *(79)* conducted a survey of pain intensity on admission and discharge from the emergency room. Highest pain intensities were caused by musculoskeletal pain in adults, but children experienced headaches as the worst pain. In addition, children who were present with only their mothers had less improvement than those who were accompanied by fathers only or both parents.

9.1.1.2. CHRONIC AND RECURRENT PAIN

Hospital admission for new-onset headache requires work-up for organic disease. Occipital neuralgia with pain over the distribution of the lesser occipital nerve is common in children with achondroplasia secondary to stenosis of the foramen magnum *(80)*.

Children with chronic pain syndromes are often admitted for acute or abortive treatment of unbearable pain, such as in intractable migraine. These acute pain episodes in the presence of chronic pain syndromes require knowledge of the chronic pain philosophies and treatment trends, as well as the armamentarium to address the patient in extreme pain. Abortive migraine treatment includes oral preparations of NSAIDs, caffeine, and isometheptene. Nausea and vomiting may require administration of intravenous antiemetics. The use of opioids or bultabital compounds is acceptable as second-line therapy, but the trend is toward using the triptan preparations *(80)* instead of narcotics. The use of ergotamines and steroids is reserved for refractory cases.

Cystic fibrosis can be associated with headaches and facial pain caused by sinusitis or coughing paroxysms *(81,82)*. Migraine and tension headaches are the most common types of pediatric headaches. By age 15 years, 5.3% of children have migraines, 15.7% have frequent nonmigrainous headaches, and 54% have infrequent nonmigrainous headaches. More than 82% of children by late adolescence experienced some type of headache *(83)*.

9.1.1.3. SICKLE CELL-RELATED PAIN

The vaso-occlusive crisis (VOC) of sickle cell disease is heralded by pain that may be localized or diffuse *(84,85)*. Sickle cell disease was first described in 1910 by Herrick *(84)*. This was the first molecular disease defined and was described by Linus Pauling *(85)*. It was Sydenstricker who first used the word *crisis* to describe the abdominal pains and jaundice that occurs during the VOC event. Ingram in 1956 examined the electrophoretic properties of normal and sickled hemoglobin and discovered the substitution of glutamic acid for valine at the sixth position of the hemoglobin chain, which led to a change in ionic charge from neutral to phobic. Deoxygenation leads to crystal formation, tactoids, and stacking of red blood cells, such that sludging in the microvasculature occurs and results in ischemia and organ infarction. Hemolysis results in jaundice *(86,87)*.

More than 2 million African Americans and Hispanic Americans are affected by sickle cell disease. Other peoples affected include those of Arab, Indian, and Asiatic descent or of descent from wherever there was malarial spread from equatorial Africa. Generally, patients present with abdominal pain, back pain, or extremity pain, especially of the legs. Any one or a combination of these regions may be affected during a VOC *(88)*. Shapiro and coworkers in the 1990s described the event as a painful episode to deemphasize the emotional component in an effort to improve coping *(89)*. Despite an attempt to control the behavioral facet by deemphasizing the anxiety, it has been shown that many patients objectively test positive for anxiety and a sense of helplessness.

Most patients with sickle cell disease have few crises that require hospitalization. Approximately only one-fourth of patients with sickle cell disease have frequent crises. Many VOC episodes are handled at home or in day hospitals, which supports the fact that early, effective intervention can curtail most uncomplicated crises *(90)*. However, when a patient fails at-home care, strong analgesics are indicated. Of patients who present to the emergency departments, 50% do so for painful events. Approximately 30% present with febrile events, and 20% come in for combined pain and fever *(91)*. Patients often require large doses of opioids but obtain minimal relief. In addition, pain scores are not inversely related to the amount of opioid administration *(92)*. Because opioids do not have a ceiling effect on analgesia, increased doses are given in an effort to decimate the pain. Often, the sedation from the opioids can be severe, resulting in inadequate ventilation, hypoxia, and worsening of the crisis pathophysiology. Acute chest syndrome, a complicated VOC presentation, has been associated with high-dose exposure to systemic opioids *(93)*.

9.1.1.4. ACUTE CANCER-RELATED PAIN

A review by Docherty found that children and adolescents with cancer focused primarily on symptoms of pain and fatigue *(94)*. Pain caused by disease occurs in fewer than 50% of cases at the time of diagnosis in pediatric oncological disease. However, children with cancer experience multiple types of pain during their course of care. Procedure-related pain because of venipunctures, bone marrow biopsies, and aspirates or lumbar punctures is common. Surgical causes of procedure-related pain include resection of solid tumors and staged procedures requiring repeated operations and placement of central intravascular access ports with subsequent removal. Some chemotherapy regimens (e.g., granulocyte-colony stimulating factor and vinca alkaloids) provoke neuropathic pain at a later time *(95)*. Organic platinum compounds such as oxaliplatin can cause pain at the onset of infusion *(96)*.

Oral mucositis results from the cytotoxic effects of chemotherapy and radiation therapy. Apoptosis of the oral epithelium occurs, and overgrowth of bacteria, fungi, and viruses in combination with the release of cytokines results in oral ulcers and a characteristic burning pain *(97)*. Resolution of the symptoms is temporally related to the recovery of the neutrophil count from the cytotoxic nadir *(98)*.

Wolfe and colleagues *(99)* found that 89% of parents felt that their children experienced "a lot" or "a great deal" from at least one symptom at the end-of-life. Pain was the most common symptom, yet only 27% of families found symptom-specific interventions to be successful in managing the pain. Parental distress can be great and is inversely proportional to the time elapsed after diagnosis *(100)*.

Death distress is usually more profound in young patients and appears to be inversely correlated to spiritual "groundedness" *(101)*. Differing spiritual beliefs between the caregiver and the adolescent patient can be a cause of worsening distress. Health professionals are encouraged to be familiar and nonjudgmental of spiritual or religious beliefs of their patients *(102)*.

The principles of cancer pain management are now well established. The Cancer Pain Relief Program of the World Health Organization developed an analgesic ladder for the management of pain of increasing intensity *(103)*. For mild pain, the recommendations start with NSAIDs. This drug class must be used with caution in those patients receiving steroids as part of their oncological management. NSAIDs are also contraindicated for patients who have renal insufficiency, intravascular volume depletion as seen with intractable vomiting, congestive heart failure, or peptic ulcer disease. A ceiling effect may occur, and increasing doses will lead to side effects without additional benefits. Unlike NSAIDs, opioids have no ceiling effect.

In the World Health Organization ladder, moderate pain is treated with traditionally weak opioids. Agents, such as codeine, oxycodone, hydrocodone, and meperidine, are used. Mixed agonists–antagonists are incorrectly considered protective against respiratory depression but may have greater side effects. These mixed agonists also have a ceiling effect. For severe pain, traditionally strong opioids are used. Unless contraindicated, morphine is generally considered the agent of choice. Other strong opioids include methadone, hydromorphone, levorphanol, and oxymorphone *(103)*.

10. Pain Intervention

10.1. Techniques

PCA is a computerized, self-administered delivery system first used in adults. Children as young as 5 years old can appropriately use the apparatus. This technique allows for single loading doses and continuous background infusions to be administered in addition to the PCA bolus dose *(104)*. The use of continuous nighttime infusions added to PCA have shown improved sleep and analgesia *(105)*. However, the use of around-the-clock, continuous background infusions have been associated with higher PCA intake *(106)*. PCA has been adapted for use by parents and caretakers for toddlers and older children who are not cognitively or physically capable of executing the self-activated PCA demand button. PCA by proxy has been administered as nurse-controlled or parent-controlled analgesia yet has been associated with a higher incidence of side effects, with oversedation the main adverse event.

In an observational study by Monitto et al., 4% of patients required naloxone reversal of sedation or apnea *(107)*. Nurse-controlled analgesia has been safely administered in children with severe cancer pain. Patients with cancer or prolonged opioid exposure may require higher infusion rates *(108)*. However, the higher the total 24-hour dose, the more likely the occurrence of side effects. Nausea and vomiting are dose-dependent and can be decreased with opioid-sparing techniques.

Epidural analgesia has been shown to provide better patient satisfaction and lower pain scores than intravenous opioid analgesia *(109,110)*. Combinations of local anesthetics with opioids or α-2 agonists provide profound analgesia with minimal sedation or respiratory depression.

Thoracic, lumbar, and sacral approaches to the epidural space have been described *(111)*. The thoracic approach via the caudal space is possible in the infant and young child because the loose areolar fat and connective tissue yield little resistance. Success in obtaining the desired level via distal entry is enhanced with nerve stimulation guidance *(112)*. The actualization of epidural anesthesia is often performed under general anesthesia. The risks of undetected nerve root trauma or spinal cord insult in the anesthetized patient is a theoretical concern. However, actualization under general anesthesia has proven to be a safe practice *(113)*. Further advances in the use of epidural and other regional techniques in children has proven to be safe and desirable for medical, perioperative, and trauma-related pain management in children.

The degree of bacterial colonization increases from the lumbar to the caudal region and poses a risk to neuraxial infection with the transfer of skin flora into the caudal space. Tunneled catheters can remain *in situ* for months without significant risk of infection *(114)*. Various barrier techniques have been tried in an effort to prevent contamination of the epidural space *(115)*. Tunneled caudal catheters reduce the risk of infection. A study by Bubeck revealed that caudal catheters that were not tunneled had three times the rate of colonization *(116)*. Peripheral nerve blocks have fewer side effects than major conduction blocks, such as epidural analgesia. However, transient nerve damage, local anesthetic toxicity, and inadequate blockade are concerns *(117–119)*. Patient-controlled regional analgesia has been reported to provide safe analgesia for postoperative pain control after lower limb surgery *(120)*.

10.1.1. Analgesics and Adjuvants

10.1.1.1. OPIOIDS

Morphine is the gold standard for strong opioids. As the prototype, *morphine equivalents* is the comparative term for converting all opioids into a user-friendly language (Table 2). The half-life of morphine is 114 minutes. Morphine sulfate (MSO_4) is metabolized by glucuronidation. Major metabolites of morphine include M-3 glucuronide, which is neutral or possibly antalgesic, and M-6-glucuronide, an active metabolite with an elimination half-life of 173 minutes *(121)*. The clearance of opioid is three to five times slower in infants younger than 3 months than in adults. Infants at 1–4 days show longer elimination half-lives than older infants (6.8 vs 3.9 hours). This difference can lead to accumulation and possibly toxic plasma levels with repeated dosing *(121,122)*. Infants older than 3 months will metabolize morphine like adults *(123)*.

Decreased responsiveness of pain to opioids may be seen in neuropathic pain because of hyperalgesia, by which the mechanism of upregulation of neurokinin-1 and substance P receptors is implicated *(124)*. G proteins form a superfamily of essential regulators that signal myriad cellular activities, including transduction, organization of the cytoskeleton, and μ opioid receptor function. Upregulation of the regulator of G protein signaling can lead to a decrease of signaling in G_i/G_o coupling of the opioid receptor *(125)*. This results in both hyperalgesia and decreased responsive to opioids. Hence, neuropathic pain can be associated with reduced opioid antinociception from multiple mechanisms. Methadone has seen resurgence because of its *N*-methyl-D-aspartate receptor antagonism because it reduces opioid tolerance and restores μ receptor activity and analgesia *(126)*.

10.1.1.2. NONSTEROIDAL ANTI-INFLAMMATORY DRUGS

NSAIDs are important to acute and chronic pain management (Table 3). The NSAIDs, when used in conjunction with opioids, are valuable in the improvement of postoperative pain by causing the opioid-sparing effects and greater reduction in pain scores *(127–129)*. The risk of perioperative bleeding does not appear

Table 3
Nonopioid Analgesics

Drug	Dose (mg/kg)	Route	Formulation	Comment
Acetaminophen	10–15 q 4 hours	po	Liquid, tablets	Limited anti-inflammatory effect
Acetyl salicylic acid	10–15 q 4 hours	po	Tablets (chewable)	Associated with Reye syndrome Antiplatelet effect, GI upset
Choline magnesium trisalicylate (Trilisate)	25 q 8–12 hours	po	Liquid, tablets	Less GI upset and antiplatelet effect than other NSAIDs
Ibuprofen	5–10 q 6 hours	po	Liquid, tablets	Antiplatelet effect, GI upset; interstitial nephritis and hepatic toxicity with chronic use
Indomethacin	1 q 8 hours	po, iv, pr	Liquid, tablet, suppository	Used in premature infants to close patent ductus arteriosus
Ketorolac	0.5 (load) 0.5 q 6 hours 10 (total dose) q 6 hours	iv, im iv, im po	Intravenous Tablets	Limit to 48–72 hours; only NSAID approved for parenteral analgesia; costly vs ibuprofen
Naproxen	5–10 q 6–8 hours	po	Liquid, tablets	*See ibuprofen*
Celecoxib	100–200 bid	po	Capsules	+ GI, – platelet effect
Rofecoxib (currently suspended)	25–50 total qd or 0.5–0.7 mg/kg	po	Suspension, tablets	– GI, – platelet effect
Tramadol	50–100 mg total per dose	po	Tablets	Some sedation, lightheadedness; per kilogram doses not available for small children

From ref. *153*. GI, gastrointestinal; NSAID, nonsteroidal anti-inflammatory drug; im, intramuscular; po, per os (by mouth); iv, intravenous.

to be affected by NSAID use *(130)*. Intravenous ketorolac has been administered after congenital heart surgery without complication.

In a study by Gupta et al., 94 children received perioperative doses of ketorolac. A relative risk of 0.2 was found for postoperative bleeding that required surgical exploration *(131)*. Neonatal dosing of ketorolac at 1 mg/kg did not cause bleeding or renal impairment. NSAIDs could prove to be efficacious in neonatal pain *(132)*.

Much attention has been given to cyclo-oxgenase (COX) inhibitors. The study of COX-1 and COX-2 isoenzymes revealed that the COX-1 isoenzyme is constitutive and continuously functioning. The COX-2 isoenzyme is inducible and is inactive in the absence of pathology. Its deleterious effects involve the inflammatory response. NSAIDs that are predominantly COX-2 inhibitors include parecoxib, valdecoxib, celecoxib, and rofecoxib.

The availability of rofecoxib as an oral suspension facilitated pediatric administration. Doses of 0.5–1.0 mg/kg up to a total dose of 50 mg were well tolerated. Children appeared to have pharmacokinetics similar to adults *(132)*. Rofecoxib was voluntarily removed from the market because of an increased incidence of cardiac and central nervous system findings in adults. No comparable untoward findings have been reported in children *(133)*. Angioedema and urticaria have occurred in isolated cases in children taking COX-2 inhibitors for rheumatological disease *(134)*.

10.1.1.3. α-2 Agonists

Clonidine, an α-2 agonist, has been administered by the oral, neuraxial, and intravenous routes for pain management in various settings. Perioperative pain control and sedation have been demonstrated by oral and rectal routes of administration *(135,136)*. Doses of 5 µg/kg are typically administered with prophylactic doses of atropine to guard against bradycardia. The literature consistently documents good pain control when clonidine is administered by the intravenous and neuraxial routes *(137,138)*.

The benefits of clonidine as an adjuvant include (1) reduction in the amount of opioid required for analgesia and thus a likely decrease in the side effects caused by opioids; (2) titrated sedation and anxiolysis without additive respiratory depression when given in combination with opioids; and (3) vasodilatation and improved circulation of cerebral, coronary, and visceral vascular beds *(139)*.

Continuous infusion of intravenous clonidine was cited in the literature approximately a decade ago as a safe adjuvant for pain control. The amount of opioids required by patients suffering procedural pain was reduced by 30%. Hemodynamic stability was maintained within normal limits as patients experienced less than a 10% change in mean blood pressure *(139)*.

The use of intravenous clonidine infusions in critically ill children has been reported as safe and efficacious without occurrence of complication or need for intervention or support because of sedation, heart rate, or blood pressure changes *(140)*.

10.1.1.4. MEMBRANE-STABILIZING AGENTS

The TCAs are used in chronic and neuropathic pain management. These cyclic amines may have intrinsic analgesic properties via cholecystokinin antagonism and may reverse established opioid tolerance *(141)*. The tertiary amines (e.g., amitriptyline) and secondary, demethylated amines (e.g., nortriptyline) have been studied more than the selective serotonin reuptake inhibitors in the treatment of neuropathic pain. TCAs are less expensive than the selective serotonin reuptake inhibitors, making the former more readily prescribed *(142)*.

Antidepressants must be taken orally for weeks to months before the onset of antinociception. When used in acute pain management, antidepressants readily improve sleep hygiene and promote restorative sleep patterns. Intravenous use of amitriptyline for acute control of mucositis pain has been cited as effective *(143)*. Cardiac rhythm changes and orthostasis can occur with intravenous amitriptyline; therefore, use in a monitored setting is encouraged *(144)*.

10.1.1.5. ANTIEPILEPTICS

AEDs are indicated for neuropathic pain. Like TCAs, delayed effect is to be expected with oral preparations. Intravenous fosphenytoin infusion for 24 hours has been purported to provide good pain relief in the case of postoperative neuroma formation *(145)*.

Generally, AEDs are prescribed for oral administration. The newer AEDs, such as gabapentin and lamotrigine, have less effect on cognitive function than carbamazepine and phenytoin. High-dose gabapentin (25–40 mg/kg/day) has been associated with aggressive behavior in children who have an underlying seizure history. Generally, gabapentin is well tolerated and is prescribed in an off-label fashion in children with neuropathic pain *(146)*. The preemptive use of gabapentin in surgical patients results in reduced opioid requirements *(147)*. AEDs may have a broader application in hospital-based pain care than is currently practiced.

11. Organizational Schemes for Hospital-Based Pain Care

There is a dearth of literature describing the current state of organized pediatric pain care in hospitals. Patient-centered care and the development of pain-free havens have been described in few US institutions *(148)*. In trying to define epidemiology and the demographics of pediatric pain services on the American continent, my colleagues and I formed a survey that examined who are the current providers, what are the services delivered, and where will organized pain services most likely be found. The unpublished 2002–2003 descriptive survey had 35. We examined the scope of practice, the subpopulation served, and the types of support given. The types of services that were provided in this country at this time appear to be interdisciplinary. Allopathic and complementary care were used in some fashion by most. More than half of the institutions possessed physician-directed pain services. Nurse-directed pain services did have a physician advisor. Physician certification in pain management was limited in pediatric pain.

The subpopulations generally served by an organized pediatric pain service are, in order of decreasing frequency, orthopedic surgery, general surgery, oncology, general pediatrics, and urological patients. More than 60% of the consultations requested were for perioperative pain care, with the remainder predominantly for medically related disease processes.

The delivery of organized hospital-based pediatric pain care likely requires an expertise that goes above and beyond that of the average requirements of a physician, nurse specialist, or other related specialists involved in clinical care. A retrospective adult study by Wheatley and coworkers showed that the incidence of postoperative chest infections decreased markedly after exposure to 1 year of acute pain service management *(149)*. More than 600 patients were treated by PCA or epidural analgesia. From 1989 to 1990, the rate of infection during the first year of the acute pain service experience decreased threefold, from 1.3 to 0.4%.

Clinically, in providing applied pharmacology and central management, it becomes clear that the pain service provider must be well versed in pain theory, pain intervention, and the impact of the pain experience. Furthermore, regardless of the institutional system of delivery of pain management services, aggressive management of the pediatric pain experience in the acute setting is critical to limit the consequences of neuroplasticity. The management of the acute pain state has been pivotal in the physiological and psychological response to future pain responses. Longitudinal and outcome studies on the efficacy of organized pediatric pain management for hospital-based pain care are needed.

References

1. IASP Task Force on Guidelines for Desirable Characteristics for Pain Treatment Facilities. Standards for Physician Fellowship in Pain Management Seattle, WA, 1990.
2. De Laat AP. Pain in Europe. IV. Fourth Congress of the European Federation of IASP Chapters (EFIC). J Orofac Pain 2004;18:69,70.

3. Stacy BR, Rudy TE, Nelhaus D. Management of patient-controlled analgesia: a comparison of primary surgeons and a dedicated pain service. Anesth Analg 1997;85:130–134.

4. Werner MU, Soholm L, Rotboll-Nielsen P, Kehlet H. Does an acute pain service improve postoperative outcome? Anesth Analg 2002;95:1361–1372.

5. Srivastava R, Homer CJ. Length of stay for common pediatric conditions: teaching vs nonteaching hospitals. Pediatrics 2003;112:278–281.

6. Fisher D, Tilford JM, Roberson PK. Relationship of illness severity and length of stay to functional outcomes in the pediatric intensive care unit: a multi-institutional study. Crit Care Med 2000;28:1173–1179.

7. Feudtner C, Christakis DA, Zimmerman FJ, Muldoon JH, Neff JM, Koepsell TD. Characteristics of deaths occurring in children's hospitals: implications for supportive care services. Pediatrics 2002;109:887–893.

8. Sakakihara Y, Yoneyama A, Kamoshita S. Chronic ventilator-assisted children in university hospitals in Japan. Acta Paediatr Jpn 1993;35:332–335.

9. Levine CD. Toxic megacolon: diagnosis and treatment challenges. AACN Clin Issues 1999;4:492–499.

10. Chiu CH, Su LH, He CC, Jaing TH, Luo CC, Lin TY. Perforation of toxic megacolon in non-typhoid *Salmonella enterocolitis* spares young infants and is immune-mediated. Pediatr Surg Int 2002;18:410–412.

11. Rees DC, Olujohungbe AD, Parker NE, Stephens AD, Telfer P, Wright J. Guidelines for the management of the acute painful crisis in sickle cell disease. Br J Haematol 2003;120:744–752.

12. Schechter NL, Allen DA, Hanson K. Status of pediatric pain control: a comparison of hospital analgesic usage in children and adults. Pediatrics 1986;77:11–15.

13. Stevens B, Hunsberger M, Browne G. Pain in children: theoretical, research and practice dilemmas. J Pediatr Nurs 1987;2:154–166.

14. Manuksela EL, Olkkala KT, Korpela R. Measurement of pain in children with self reporting and behavioral assessment. Clin Pharmacol Ther 1987;42:37–41.

15. Fradet C, McGrath PJ, Kay J, Adams S, Luke B. A prospective survey of reactions to blood tests by children and adolescents. Pain 1990;40:53–60.

16. Shapiro RS. Health care providers' liability exposure for inappropriate pain management. J Law Med Ethics 1996;24:360–364.

17. Donovan M, Dillon P, McGuire L. Incidence and characteristics of pain in a sample of medical-surgical inpatients. Pain 1987;30:69–78.

18. Rennick J, Johnston CC, Dougherty G, Platt R, Ritchie J. Children's psychological responses after critical illness and exposure to invasive technology. J Dev Behav Pediatr 2002;23:133–144.

19. Saxe G, Stoddard F, Courtney D, et al. Relationship between acute morphine and the course of PTSD in children with burns. J Am Acad Child Adolesc Psychiatry 2001;40:915–921.

20. Taddio A, Shah V, Gilbert-MacLeod C, Katz J. Conditioning and hyperalgesia in newborns exposed to repeated heel lances. JAMA 2002;288:857–861.

21. Taddio A, Katz J, Ilersich AL, Lane A, Koren G. Effect of neonatal circumcision on pain response during subsequent routine vaccination. Lancet 1997;349:599–603.

22. Andrews K, Fitzgerald M. Barriers to optimal pain management in infants, children and adolescents: biological barriers to paediatric pain management. Clin J Pain 1997;13:138–143.
23. Beeson JM. The neurobiology of pain. Lancet 1999;353:1610–1615.
24. Fitzgerald M, Jennings E. The postnatal development of spinal sensory processing. Proc Natl Acad Sci USA 1999;96:7719–7722.
25. Marsh DF, Hatch DJ, Fitzgerald M. Opioid systems and the newborn. Br J Anaesth 1997;79:787–795.
26. Turk DC, Okifuji A. Pain terms and taxonomies of pain In: Loeser JD, ed. Bonica's Management of Pain. 3rd ed. Philadelphia: Lippincott, Williams, and Wilkins; 2001:17–25.
27. Anand KJS, Hickey PR. Pain and its effects in the human neonate and fetus. N Engl J Med 1987;317:1321–1329.
28. Perl ER. Cutaneous polymodal receptors: characteristics and plasticity. Prog Brain Res 1996;113:21–28.
29. Mense S. Group III and IV receptors in skeletal muscle: are they specific or polymodal? Prog Brain Res 1996;113:85–100.
30. Cervero F, Lumb BM. Bilateral inputs and supraspinal control of viscero-somatic neurons in the lower thoracic spinal cord of the cat. J Physiol 1988;403:221–237.
31. Mayer EA, Gebhart GF. Basic and clinical aspects of visceral hyperalgesia. Gastroenterology 1994;107:271–293.
32. Garry EM, Moss A, Rosie R, Delaney A, Mitchell R, Fleetwood-Walker SM. Specific involvement in neuropathic pain of AMPA receptors and adapter proteins for the GluR2 subunit. Mol Cell Neurosci 2003;24:10–22.
33. Fitzgerald M, Jennings E. The postnatal development of spinal sensory processing. Proc Natl Acad Sci USA 1999;96:7719–7722.
34. Gunnar MR, Porter FL, Wolf CM, Rigatuso J, Larson MC. Neonatal stress reactivity: predictions to later emotional temperament. Child Dev 1995;66:1–13.
35. Dubin AE, Dionne VE. Action potentials and chemosensitive conductances in the dendrites of olfactory neurons suggest new features for odor transduction. J Gen Physiol 1994;103:181–201.
36. Traub RJ. Spinal modulation of the induction of central sensitization. Brain Res 1997;778:34–42.
37. Millan MJ. The induction of pain: an integrative review. Prog Neurobiol 1999;57:1–164.
38. Lugo RA, Kern SE. Clinical pharmacokinetics of morphine. J Pain Palliat Care Pharmacother 2002;16:5–18.
39. Belpaire FM, Bogaert MG. Binding of alfentanil to human α1-acid glycoprotein, albumin and serum. Int J Clin Pharmacol Ther Toxicol 1991;29:96–102.
40. Sutton SC. Companion animal physiology and dosage form performance. Adv Drug Deliv Rev 2004;56:1383–1398.
41. deBoer AG, Moolenaar F, deLeede LG, Breimer DD. Rectal drug administration: clinical pharmacokinetic considerations. Clin Pharmacokinet 1982;7:285–311.
42. Lesser E, Chhabra R, Brion LP, Suresh BR. Use of midline catheters in low birth weight infants. J Perinatol 1996;16(3, pt 1):205–207.

43. Carr DB, Jacox AK, Chapman CR, et al. Acute pain management: Operative or Medical Procedures and Trauma. Clinical Practice Guideline. Rockville, MD: Agency for Health Care Policy and Research, Public Health Service, US Dept of Health and Human Services; 1992. AHCPR Pub. No. 92-0032.

44. Edwards WT. Optimizing opioid treatment of postoperative pain. J Pain Symptom Manage 1990;5(suppl. 1):S24–S36.

45. Lewis N. The needle is like an animal: how children view injections. Child Today 1978;7:18–21.

46. Mathew PJ, Mathew JL. Assessment and management of pain in infants. Postgrad Med J 2003;79:438–443.

47. Bray RJ, Beeton C, Hinton W, Seviour JA. Plasma morphine levels produced by continuous infusion in children. Anaesthesia 1986;41:753–755.

48. Kehlet H, Dahl JB. The value of "multimodal" or "balanced analgesia" in postoperative pain treatment. Anesth Analg 1993;77:1048–1056.

49. Ramsay MAE. Acute postoperative pain management BUMC Proc 2000;13: 244–247.

50. Fitzgibbon DR. Cancer pain: management. In: Loeser JD, ed. Bonica's Management of Pain. 3rd ed. Philadelphia: Lippincott, Williams, and Wilkins; 2001, pp. 661–703.

51. Ready LB. Regional analgesia with intraspinal opioids. In: Loeser JD, ed. Bonica's Management of Pain. 3rd ed. Philadelphia: Lippincott, Williams, and Wilkins; 2001, pp. 1953–1966.

52. Ivanenko A, Tauman R, Gozal D. Modafinil in the treatment of excessive daytime sleepiness in children. Sleep Med 2003;4:579–582.

53. Besset A, Chetrit M, Carlander B, Billiard M. Use of modafinil in the treatment of narcolepsy: a long term follow-up study. Neurophysiol Clin 1996;26:60–66.

54. Ready LB, Edwards WT. The Management of Acute Pain: Practical Guidelines. Seattle, WA: IASP Press; 1992, pp. 1–79.

55. Kain ZN, Caramico LA, Mayes LC, Genevro JL, Bornstein MH, Hofstadter MB. Preoperative preparation programs in children: a comparative examination. Anesth Analg 1998;87:1249–1255.

56. Kain ZN, Caldwell-Andrews AA, Maranets I, et al. Preoperative anxiety and emergence delirium and postoperative maladaptive behaviors. Anesth Analg 2004; 99:1648–1654.

57. Katz J. Pre-emptive analgesia: importance of timing. Can J Anesth 2001;48: 105–114.

58. McQuay HJ. Effectiveness of pre-emptive analgesia: a systematic review of clinical studies. Ann Med 1995;27:249–256.

59. Willard PT, Blair NP. Is wound infiltration with anesthetic effective as pre-emptive analgesia? A clinical trial in appendectomy patients. Can J Surg 1997;40:213–217.

60. Ho JW, Khambatta HJ, Pang LM, Siegfried RN, Sun LS. Preemptive analgesia in children. Does it exist? Reg Anesth 1997;22:125–130.

61. Priya V, Divatia JV, Sareen R, Upadhye S. Efficacy of intravenous ketoprofen for pre-emptive analgesia. J Postgrad Med 2002;48:109–112.

62. Park J, Forrest J, Kolesar R, et al. Oral clonidine reduces postoperative PCA morphine requirements. Can J Anaesth 1996;43:900–906.
63. Goyagi T, Tanaka M, Nishikawa T. Oral clonidine premedication enhances postoperative analgesia by epidural morphine. Anesth Analg 1999;89:1487–1491.
64. Kain ZN, Sevarino F, Pincus S, et al. Attenuation of the preoperative stress response with midazolam: effects on postoperative outcomes. Anesthesiology 2000;93: 141–147.
65. Puncuh F, Lampugnani E, Kokki H. Use of spinal anaesthesia in paediatric patients: a single centre experience with 1132 cases. Paediatr Anaesth 2004;14:564–567.
66. Portenoy RK, Hagen NA. Breakthrough pain: definition and management. Oncology (Huntingt) 1989;3(8 suppl):25–29.
67. Svendsen KB, Andersen S, Arnason S, et al. Breakthrough pain in malignant and non-malignant diseases: a review of prevalence, characteristics and mechanisms. Eur J Pain 2005;9:195–206.
68. Caraceni A, Martini C, Zecca E, et al. Working Group of an IASP Task Force on Cancer Pain. Breakthrough pain characteristics and syndromes in patients with cancer pain. An international survey. Palliat Med 2004;18:177–183.
69. Gallagher SS, Finison K, Guyer B, Goodenough S. The incidence of injuries among 87,000 Massachusetts children and adolescents: results of the 1980–81 statewide Childhood Injury Prevention Program Surveillance System. Am J Public Health 1984;74:1340–1347.
70. Martinez-Herz SP, Patterson DR, Honari S. Pediatric pain control practices of North American Burn Centers. J Burn Care Rehabil 2003;24:26–36.
71. Huribal M, Cunningham ME, D'Aiuto ML. Endothelin-1 and prostaglandin E2 levels increase in patients with burn. J Am Coll Surg 1995;180:318–322.
72. Kowalske KJ, Tanelian D. Burn pain, evaluation and management. Anesthesiol Clin North Am 1997;15:269–283.
73. Kinsella J, Booth M. Pain relief in burns: James Laing memorial essay 1990. Burns 1991;17:391–395.
74. Treede RD, Meyer RA, Raja SN, et al. Peripheral and central mechanisms of cutaneous hyperalgesia. Prog Neurobiol 1992;38:397–421.
75. Ashburn M. Burn pain: The management of procedure related burn. J Burn Care Rehabil 1995;16:365–371.
76. Martinez-Herz SP, Thurber CA, Patterson DR. Psychological principles of burn wound pain in children. II: Treatment applications. J Burn Care Rehabil 2000;21: 458–472.
77. Thurber CA, Martinez-Herz SP, Patterson DR. Psychological principles of burn wound pain in children. I: Theoretical framework. J Burn Care Rehabil 2000;1: 376–387.
78. Galustyan S, Kim M, Sato TA, Hennes H. Analgesia for children with acute abdominal pain. Acad Emerg Med 2002;9:522.
79. Johnston CC, Gagnon AJ, Fullerton L, Common C, Ladores M, Forlini S. One-wk survey of pain intensity on admission to and discharge from the emergency department: a pilot study. J Emerg Med 1998;16:377–382.

80. Kondev L, Minster A. Headache and facial pain in children and adolescents. Otolaryngol Clin North Am 2003;6:1153–1170.

81. Marks SC, Kissner DG. Management of sinusitis in adult cystic fibrosis. Am J Rhinol 1997;11:11–14.

82. Stern RC, Horowitz SJ, Doershuk CF. Neurologic symptoms during coughing paroxysms in cystic fibrosis. J Pediatr 1988;112:909–912.

83. Lipton RB. Diagnosis and epidemiology of pediatric migraine. Curr Opin Neurol 1997;10:231.

84. Herrick JB. Peculiar elongated and sickle-shaped red blood corpuscles in a case of severe anemia. Arch Intern Med 1910;6:517–521.

85. Pauling L. The normal hemoglobins and the hemoglobinopathies: background. Tex Rep Biol Med 1980;81;40:1–7.

86. Ballas SK. Sickle cell anaemia: progress in pathogenesis and treatment. Drugs 2002;62:1143–1172.

87. Wethers DL. Sickle cell disease in childhood: Part I. Laboratory diagnosis, pathophysiology and health maintenance. Am Fam Physician 2000;62:1013–1020.

88. Serjeant GR, Serjeant BE. Sickle cell disease in Saudi Arabia: the Asian haplotype. Reflections on a meeting at Hofuf, September 2003. Ann Saudi Med 2004;24: 166–168.

89. Shapiro BS, Dinges DF, Orne EC, et al. Home management of sickle cell-related pain in children and adolescents: natural history and impact on school attendance. Pain 1995;61:139–144.

90. Benjamin LJ, Swinson GI, Nagel RL. Sickle cell anemia day hospital: an approach for the management of uncomplicated painful crises. Blood 2000;95: 1130–1136.

91. Frush K, Ware RE, Kinney TR. Emergency department visits by children with sickle hemoglobinopathies: factors associated with hospital admission. Pediatr Emerg Care 1995;11:9–12.

92. Jacob E, Miaskowski C, Savedra M, Beyer JE, Treadwell M, Styles L. Management of vaso-occlusive pain in children with sickle cell disease. Am J Pediatr Hematol Oncol 2003;25:307–311.

93. Kopecky EA, Jacobson S, Joshi P, Koren G. Systemic exposure to morphine and the risk of acute chest syndrome in sickle cell disease. Clin Pharmacol Ther 2004;75:140–146.

94. Docherty SL. Symptom experiences of children and adolescents with cancer. Annu Rev Nurs Res 2003;21:123–149.

95. Topp KS, Tanner KD, Levine JD. Damage to the cytoskeleton of large diameter sensory neurons and myelinated axons in vincristine-induced painful peripheral neuropathy in the rat. J Comp Neurol 2000;424:563–576.

96. Quasrhoff S, Hartung HP. Chemotherapy-induced peripheral neuropathy. J Neurol 2002;249:9–17.

97. Köstler WJ, Hejna M, Wenzel C, Zielinski CC. Oral mucositis complicating chemotherapy and/or radiotherapy: options for prevention and treatment. CA Cancer J Clin 2001;51:290–315.

98. Lockhart PB, Sonis ST. Relationship of oral complications to peripheral blood leukocyte and platelet counts in patients receiving cancer chemotherapy. Oral Surg Oral Med Oral Pathol 1979;48:21–28.

99. Wolfe J, Grier HE, Klar N, et al. Symptoms and suffering at the end of life in children with cancer. N Engl J Med 2000;342:326–333.

100. Boman K, Lindahl A, Bjork O. Disease-related distress in parents of children with cancer at various stages after the time of diagnosis. Acta Oncol 2003;42: 137–146.

101. Chibnall JT, Videen SD, Duckro PN, Miller DK. Psychosocial-spiritual correlates of death distress in patients with life-threatening medical conditions. Palliat Med 2002;16:331–338.

102. Lyon ME, Townsend-Akpan C, Thompson A. Spirituality and end-of-life care for an adolescent with AIDS. Aids Patient Care Stds 2001;15:555–560.

103. Jacox AK, Carr DB, Payne R, et al. Management of Cancer Pain: Clinical Practice Guideline. Rockville, MD: Agency for Health Care Policy and Research, Public Health Service, US Department of Health and Human Services; 1994. AHCPR Pub. No. 94-0592.

104. McDonald AJ, Cooper MG. Patient-controlled analgesia: an appropriate method of pain control in children. Paediatr Drugs 2001;3:273–284.

105. Doyle E, Robinson D, Morton NS. Comparison of patient-controlled analgesia with and without a background infusion after lower abdominal surgery in children. Br J Anaesth 1993;71:670–673.

106. Yildiz K, Tercan E, Dogru K, Ozkan U, Boyaci A. Comparison of patient-controlled analgesia with and without a background infusion after appendectomy in children. Paediatr Anaesth 2003;13:427–431.

107. Monitto CL, Greenberg RS, Kost-Byerly S, et al. The safety and efficacy of parent-/nurse-controlled analgesia in patients less than 6 yr of age. Anesth Analg 2000; 91:573–579.

108. McDonald AJ, Cooper MG. Patient-controlled analgesia: an appropriate method of pain control in children. Paediatr Drugs 2001;3:273–284.

109. Bai SJ, Koo BN, Kim JH, Doh PS, Kim KH, Shin YS. Comparison of continuous epidural and intravenous analgesia for postoperative pain control in pediatric lower extremity surgery. Yonsei Med J 2004;45:789–795.

110. Blumenthal S, Min K, Nadig M, Borgeat A. Double epidural catheter with ropivacaine vs intravenous morphine: a comparison for postoperative analgesia after scoliosis correction surgery. Anesthesiology 2005;102:175–180.

111. Tsui BC, Wagner A, Cave D, Kearney R. Thoracic and lumbar epidural analgesia via the caudal approach using electrical stimulation guidance in pediatric patients: a review of 289 patients. Anesthesiology 2004;100:683–689.

112. Tsui BC, Seal R, Entwistle L, Haugen R, Kearney R. Thoracic epidural analgesia via the caudal approach in pediatric patients undergoing fundoplication using nerve stimulation guidance. Anesth Analg 2001;93:1152–1155.

113. Krane EJ, Dalens BJ, Murat I, Murrell D. The safety of epidurals placed during general anesthesia. Reg Anesth Pain Med 1998;23:433–438.

114. Aram L, Krane EJ, Kozloski LJ, Yaster M. Tunneled epidural catheters for prolonged analgesia in pediatric patients. Anesth Analg 2001;92:1432–1438.

115. McClain BC, Redd SA. Barrier flaps for continuous caudal anesthesia in pediatric patients. Anesthesiology 1993;79:400–401.

116. Bubeck J, Boos K, Krause H, Thies KC. Subcutaneous tunneling of caudal catheters reduces the rate of bacterial colonization to that of lumbar epidural catheters. Anesth Analg 2004;99:689–693.

117. Berde C. Regional anesthesia in children: what have we learned? Anesth Analg 1996;83:897–900.

118. Johnson CM. Continuous femoral nerve blockade for analgesia in children with femoral fractures. Anaesth Intensive Care 1994;22:281–283.

119. Maccani RM, Wedel DJ, Melton A, Gronert GA. Femoral and lateral femoral cutaneous nerve block for muscle biopsies in children. Paediatr Anaesth 1995;5: 223–227.

120. Duflo F, Qamouss Y, Remond C, et al. Patient-controlled regional analgesia is effective in children: a preliminary report. Can J Anaesth 2004;51:928–930.

121. Tyler DC. Pharmacology of pain management. Pediatr Clin North Am 1994;41: 59–71.

122. Lynn AM, Slattery JT. Morphine pharmacokinetics in early infancy. Anesthesiology 1987;66:136–139.

123. Berde CB. Pediatric postoperative pain management. Pediatr Clin North Am 1989;36:921–940.

124. Velazquez RA, McCarson KE, Cai Y, et al. Upregulation of neurokinin-1 receptor of expression in rat spinal cord by an N-terminal metabolite of substance P. Eur J Neurosci 2002;16:229–241.

125. Garnier M, Zaratin PF, Ficalora G, et al. Up-regulation of regulator of G-protein signaling 4 expression in a model of neuropathic pain and insensitivity to morphine. J Pharmacol Exp Ther 2003;304:1299–1306.

126. Morley JS, Bridson J, Nash T, Miles JB, White S, Makin MK. Low dose methadone has an analgesic effect in neuropathic pain: a double- blind randomized controlled crossover trial. Palliat Med 2003;17:576–587.

127. Miller OF, Bloom TL, Smith LJ, McAleer IM, Kaplan GW, Kolon TF. Early hospital discharge for intravesical ureteroneocystostomy. J Urol 2002;167:2556–2559.

128. Nishina K, Mikawa K, Shiga M, Takao Y, Maekawa N, Obara H. Diclofenac and flurbiprofen with or without clonidine for postoperative analgesia in children undergoing elective ophthalmological surgery. Paediatr Anaesth 2000;10:645–651.

129. Romsing J, Ostergaard D, Walther-Larsen S, Valentin N. Analgesic efficacy and safety of preoperative vs postoperative ketorolac in psediatric tonsillectomy. Acta Anaesthesiol Scand 1998;42:770–775.

130. Romsing J, Walther-Larsen S. Perioperative use of nonsteroidal anti-inflammatory drugs in children: analgesic efficacy and bleeding. Anaesthesia 1997;52:673–683.

131. Gupta A, Daggett C, Ludwick J, Wells W, Lewis LA. Ketorolac after congenital heart surgery: does it increase the risk of significant bleeding complications? Paediatr Anaesth 2005;15:139–142.

132. Papacci P, De Francissi G, Iacobucci T, et al. Use of intravenous ketorolac in the neonate and premature babies. Paediatr Anaesth 2004;14:487–492.

133. Prescilla RP, Frattarelli DA, Haritos D, Aranda JV, Edwards DJ. Pharmacokinetics of rofecoxib in children with sickle cell hemoglobinopathy. J Pediatr Hematol Oncol 2004;26:661–664.

134. Kamen B, Kieran M. Don't throw out the baby with the bathwater! J Pediatr Hematol Oncol 2005;27:59–60.

135. Bergendahl HT, Lonnqvisy PA, Eksborg S, et al. Clonidine vs midazolam as premediciation in children undergoing adeno-tonsillectomy: a prospective, randomized, controlled clinical trial. Acta Anaesthesiol Scand 2004;48:1292–1300.

136. Broadman LM, Rice LJ, Hannallah RS. Oral clonidine and postoperative pain. Anesth Analg 1996;82:225–230.

137. Sung CS, Lin SH, Chan KH, et al. Effect of oral clonidine premedication on perioperative hemodynamic response and postoperative analgesic requirements for patients undergoing laparoscopic cholecystectomy. Acta Anaesthesiol Sin 2000;38:23–29.

138. Lyons B, Casey W, Doherty P, McHugh M, Moore KP. Pain relief with low-dose intravenous clonidine in a child with severe burns. Intensive Care Med 1996;22: 249–251.

139. Eisenach JC, De Kock M, Klimscha W. $\alpha(2)$-Adrenergic agonists for regional anesthesia. A clinical review of clonidine (1984–1995). Anesthesiology 1996;85: 655–674.

140. Ambrose C, Sale S, Howells R, et al. Intravenous clonidine infusion in critically ill children: dose-dependent sedative effects and cardiovascular stability. Br J Anaesth 2000;84:794–796.

141. Coudore-Civiale MA, Courteix C, Boucher M. Potentiation of morphine and clomipramine analgesia by cholecystokinin B antagonist CI 988 in diabetic rats. Neurosci Lett 2000;286:37–40.

142. Stacey BR. Management of peripheral neuropathic pain. Am J Phys Rehabil 2005;84(3 suppl):S4–S16.

143. Collins JJ, Kerner J, Sentivany S, Berde CB. Intravenous amitriptyline in pediatrics. J Pain Symptom Manage 1995;10:471–475.

144. Donmez O, Cetinkaya M, Canbek R. Hemoperfusion in a child with amitriptyline intoxication. Pediatr Nephrol 2005;20:105–107.

145. Tallian KB, Nahata MC, Lo W, Tsao CY. Gabapentin associated with aggressive behavior in pediatric patients with seizures. Epilepsia 1996;37:501–502.

146. McGraw T, Stacey BR. Gabapentin for treatment of neuropathic pain in a 12-yr-old girl. Clin J Pain 1998;14:354–356.

147. Gilron I, Orr E, Tu D, O'Neill JP, Zamora JE, Bell AC. A placebo-controlled randomized clinical trial of perioperative administration of gabapentin, rofecoxib and their combination for spontaneous and movement-evoked pain after abdominal hysterectomy. Pain 2005;113:191–200.

148. Schechter NL, Blankson V, Pachter LM, Sullivan CM, Costa L. The ouchless place: no pain, children's gain. Pediatrics 1997;99:890–894.

149. Wheatley RG, Madej TH, Jackson IJ, Hunter D. The first year's experience of an acute pain service. Br J Anaesth 1991;67:353–359.
150. Guyton AC, Hall JE, eds. Textbook of Medical Physiology. 10th ed. Philadelphia: Saunders; 2000;512–565.
151. Pereira J, Lawlor P, Vigano A, Dorgan M, Bruera E. Equianalgesic dose ratios for opioids. A critical review and proposals for long-term dosing. J Pain Symptom Manage 2001;22:672–687.
152. Anderson R, Saiers JH, Abram S, Schlicht C. Accuracy in equianalgesic dosing: conversion dilemmas. J Pain Symptom Manage 2001;21:397–406.
153. McClain BC. Yale New Haven Children's Hospital Pediatric Pain Service Postgraduate Guide. New Haven, CT: Yale New Haven Children's Hospital, Department of Anesthesiology; 2001.

2

Treatment of Acute and Chronic Pain in the Outpatient Setting

Neil L. Schechter

Summary

Although there have been dramatic changes in attitude and practice in the treatment of children's pain in the hospital, pain management in outpatient settings is treated essentially the way it was 20 years ago. It is quite remarkable that many common illnesses and procedures universally acknowledged to be associated with significant discomfort and anxiety have received minimal research attention. In this chapter, some of the more common pain problems (minor procedures and acute illnesses) encountered in office practice are reviewed, and suggestions for pain relief based on the limited literature are offered. The following areas are addressed: (1) pain associated with immunization, the most common painful procedure in office practice; (2) pain associated with common illnesses, specifically otitis media, pharyngitis, and viral mouth infections; and (3) chronic and recurrent pains, which require an alternative paradigm than acute pain. Through the uniform use of relatively simple strategies, much of the pain associated with these common problems can be significantly reduced.

Key Words: Chronic pain; immunization; otitis media, pharyngitis.

1. Introduction

The past 20 years have been witness to a revolution in the way pain is conceptualized and managed in children. This change is most evident in the treatment of hospitalized children with significant pain problems. The treatment of postoperative pain, for example, is dramatically different from what it was two decades ago, when it was essentially ignored or at best addressed haphazardly *(1)*. The outpouring of research attention that has been given to this problem coupled with the recognition that untreated pain may have negative consequences for the child *(2,3)* has been largely responsible for this change in practice. Similar attention has also been focused on cancer pain *(4,5)* and pain in the

From: *Bringing Pain Relief to Children: Treatment Approaches*
Edited by: G. A. Finley, P. J. McGrath, and C. T. Chambers © Humana Press Inc., Totowa, NJ

newborn nursery *(6,7)*, and the treatment of these problems has likewise improved significantly. Policies and procedures are in place in most centers that care for children to ensure that hospitalized children with predictable pain problems such as those mentioned receive appropriate care.

This change in practice, however, for the most part remains limited to treatment in the hospital. Remarkably, pain management in children in ambulatory settings is treated essentially the same way it was 20 years ago. This is all the more striking given the frequency of these pain problems compared with those associated with hospitalization. For example, there is almost no research addressing pain in otitis media or pharyngitis, which are often associated with significant distress and are among the most common causes of childhood visits to the physician. The pain associated with immunizations is another example. There are literally hundreds of millions of immunizations given yearly to children in physician offices and clinics around the world. For many children, these injections are so stressful that they color the child's entire relationship with his or her health care provider. Yet, the paucity of data on strategies that might alleviate some of the discomfort associated with them is quite remarkable. Likewise, common chronic pains, such as headache, abdominal pain, and limb pain, although subjected to some academic scrutiny, have yielded no uniformly accepted approach to their evaluation or treatment.

There are a variety of reasons for this lack of interest in these common pain problems. First, they are far less dramatic than the problems of children with life-threatening illness. Studying the pain of a self-limited illness like otitis media or a minor procedure like an immunization lacks the cachet, poignancy, and sense of urgency that exists for pain problems in the hospital. Chronic pain problems are often seen as vague and multifactorial, and as a result do not lend themselves to simple solutions; therefore, they are often perceived as both time consuming and nonrewarding for the physician. Significantly as well, there are limited financial incentives in this market for the pharmaceutical industry. Research on children is costly and fraught with ethical complexities. Because many of these problems are not seen as pressing and because drugs developed will have only short-term use, this market is felt to be limited. As a result, there has been little investigation into the treatment of these frequently encountered problems. The disparity between the frequency with which these pains are encountered and the paucity of research regarding them will become evident to the reader. This lack of investigation and interest, however, does not mitigate the fact that these problems impose a significant burden on children.

Commonly encountered pains in ambulatory settings can typically be categorized as acute or chronic. In the category of acute pain, there are the normative pains of childhood (teething); the pains associated with infection (such as otitis media, pharyngitis, viral infections of the mouth, and urinary tract infections);

the pain associated with minor procedures, such as injections, phlebotomy, urinary catheterization, and laceration repair; and pain associated with minor musculoskeletal injury, such as strains and sprains. Chronic or recurrent pains are defined as pain occurring either persistently or at least three times over the course of 3 months *(8)*. These include headache, recurrent abdominal pain, limb and back pain, widespread musculoskeletal pain, such as fibromyalgia, or pain that does not seem to remit associated with minor injury, such as reflex sympathetic dystrophy.

This chapter obviously cannot address this extensive list but attempts to review a number of the major common pains encountered in pediatric outpatient settings. In particular, the discussion focuses primarily on immunization pain, an area not been comprehensively reviewed in the past, selected infection-related pains, and a general overview of chronic pain in children.

2. Acute Pain

2.1. Immunizations

Immunizations are the most frequently occurring painful procedure in pediatric settings. These procedures have an enormous positive impact on disease prevention. For example, prior to the development of vaccines, there were 170,000 cases of diphtheria, 16,000 cases of paralytic poliomyelitis, and 500,000 cases of measles reported annually. In 2001, there were 2 cases of diphtheria, no cases of polio, and 116 cases of measles *(9)*. It is obvious that the impact of these agents on reducing the burden of disease is almost incalculable. There has been steady growth in the number of immunizations given to children and adults. At the present time, according to the most recent immunization schedule, more than 20 immunizations are given to children by the age of 2 years and more than 26 throughout childhood. The sheer volume of immunizations has necessitated that multiple injections must be given at a health supervision visit. For example, at the typical 2-month visit, up to five separate immunizations may be given. At the 4-month visit, four immunizations may be given; at the 6-month visit, about five immunizations may be given *(10)*.

Despite their undeniable value, these procedures are a mixed blessing. On the one hand, they protect the children from life-threatening illnesses. On the other hand, all health care providers who work with children are familiar with the anxiety that the anticipation of these procedures engenders. Every nurse or physician who works with children has entered the examining room and encountered a worried child cringing in the corner whose first question is, "Am I going to get a shot?" For a subset of children, the concerns about these procedures dominate the entire encounter with their health care provider. Preoccupation with these procedures affects not only the child, however, but also has a significant impact on families and on the health care provider.

2.1.1. Impact of Immunization Pain on the Child

The impact of the immunization on the child is intuitive and obvious. In multiple studies *(11,12)*, the needle has been shown to be the most powerful negative symbol associated with medical care. Needle phobia is a well-established concern among many children. We now also know, that during infancy children have memory for pain and can anticipate painful procedures if they have experienced them recently *(13)*. Research has also suggested that children react more intensely to new procedures if they have had previous painful procedures without adequate anesthesia. This has been demonstrated with circumcisions *(14)*, painful procedures in the newborn intensive care unit *(15)*, and bone marrow aspirations in older children *(16)*. We also know that there is a wide variation of response to injections among different children and even at different times in the same child.

In an attempt to understand the individual differences among children in response to injections, we studied the impact of a host of variables on the children's response to their 5-year preschool injection *(17)*. At a home visit 1 month prior to the scheduled injection, parents were queried regarding their own attitudes toward pain, their personal experiences with pain, and their child-rearing attitudes. A questionnaire categorizing the child's temperament was also given to parents. Finally, they were asked to predict the degree of distress they felt their child would experience during the injection. Children were also interviewed in an attempt to assess the degree of anxiety about the pending immunization they were experiencing. At the visit to the medical office 1 month later, the child's response to the immunization was assessed using their self-report on the Oucher *(18)*, as well as Visual Analog Scale (VAS) ratings by the parent and provider. In addition, the Procedure Rating Scale *(19)*, which assesses "pain behaviors" was also administered.

This study identified a subset of children—perhaps 10–15%—who displayed significant distress at the procedure and who rated the pain associated with the immunization as "the most pain imaginable." Surprisingly, parental characteristics and attributes did not predict children who experienced the most distress. The strongest predictor was the parent's rating of the child's temperament. In particular, children who have more "difficult" temperamental styles have more distress. The trait of adaptability correlated most strongly with distress: the less adaptable, the more distressed. Also, parents were able to predict how their child would react to the injection. Others *(20,21)* also identified the important role of temperament in defining children's response to painful procedures.

2.1.2. Impact of Immunization Pain on the Family

It is not only the child who is concerned about immunization pain. Meyerhoff et al. *(22)* attempted to quantify parental concern about immunization pain using a methodology entitled *willingness to pay*. Their group asked families how much they would be willing to pay to eliminate the discomfort associated with immunization pain. Parents, regardless of socioeconomic level, stated that they would pay "on average" $57 to eliminate the pain of a two-shot visit and $80 to eliminate the pain of a three-shot visit. Regardless of the specific numeric value and whether, in fact, parents would actually pay the amount they implied they would, this study clearly suggested that parents have concerns about the distress associated with immunization and desired, if possible, to ameliorate some of that discomfort.

There is other evidence that parents have significant concerns about immunization pain. Reis *(23)* suggested that parental concern about injections may well have an impact on their compliance with medical care in infancy. New work using functional magnetic resonance imaging (fMRI) technology supports the depth of parental distress. Singer et al. *(24)* proposed the notion of pain empathy. They examined fMRI data in individuals experiencing pain and compared that with fMRIs of those individuals when witnessing a loved one experience pain. They found that the structures involved in the emotional aspect of pain (the bilateral anterior insula, rostral anterior cingulate cortex, brain stem, and cerebellum) were activated similarly both in individuals who were subjected to painful experiences and in those who were witnessing a loved one being subjected to a painful experience. The emotional aspect of pain was identical in both individuals. The brain structures associated directly with the sensory experience of pain (posterior insula, somatosensory and sensorimotor cortex, as well as the caudal interior cingulate cortex) were only activated in the individuals who were directly subjected to the painful experience. They interpreted this data to suggest that the response of an individual observing a loved one experience pain was almost identical to the emotional aspect of pain in the individual receiving it. Certainly, the case can be made that parents experience profound emotional distress when witnessing their child experience the discomfort of an immunization, especially because they are helpless to protect the child from this pain or to ameliorate it once it has occurred.

2.1.3. Impact of Immunization Pain on the Provider

Not only the parents and the child are distressed by the pain associated with immunizations; the health care provider is distressed as well. Woodin et al. *(25)* evaluated the impact on providers of giving multiple injections. In an article, "Are Children Becoming Pincushions?," they identified that 65% of physicians reported strong concerns about administering four injections to infants at one visit. More than 80% of physicians had strong concerns about giving multiple injections in general. In fact, physicians were more likely to be troubled than parents about the number of shots that they are expected to administer under the current immunization schedule. Reis *(26)* reported that physicians were six times less likely to give all the immunizations at a visit if three or more were scheduled than if two or fewer were scheduled.

It is obvious, therefore, that children, parents, and health care providers all have strong concerns about the pain engendered by immunizations. Despite this concern and the frequency with which immunizations are administered, there has been strikingly little research on reducing immunization pain. Although the literature is limited, the following components of injection pain are reviewed: prior to the injection (these are preparation and education), selection of the appropriate site and needle gage, and injectate properties and administration technique; during the injection, we review securing the child, use of nonpharmacological strategies, local anesthetic, and physical approaches.

2.1.4. Prior to the Immunization

2.1.4.1. PREPARATION

Preparation of the child and his or her family is an essential aspect of pain reduction. If parents are less anxious, they can convey that to the child, which may have a positive impact on the child's perception of the painful stimulus. There is a well-established relationship between anxiety and increased pain perception. Parents should be informed of the reason for the injection and its potential value to their child. There should be realistic discussion about the pain associated with it and the potential complications of the injection. Parents should be queried regarding their perception of their child's coping style (information seeking or avoidant). This may help the provider in subsequent discussions with the child. Finally, parents of toddlers, preschoolers, and school-aged children should be offered some distraction techniques that they can use for this and for subsequent procedures. These may include reading or telling favorite stories, breathing, and blowing techniques.

Regarding preparation of the child, there is amazingly limited research available to guide practice. Obviously, the type and extent of preparation should be based on the child's age and developmental level. In general, content has more relevance for children over the age of 2 years. Toddlers and preschoolers should be informed of the procedure as close to the time it will occur as possible. Most authorities suggest that preparation for all procedures should include at least two elements *(27,28)*: (1) what will happen (that is, what exactly will be done, how long it will take, etc.) and (2) how it will feel (i.e., the coolness of the alcohol swab, the pinch of the needle, etc.). It also may help for children to be asked what strategies they believe will help them effectively deal with the procedure.

2.1.4.2. SELECTING THE APPROPRIATE SITE

In general, there appears to be some agreement regarding the site at which intramuscular injections should be administered. Consensus statements from major professional and educational organizations suggest that the anterior lateral thigh should be used in infants, and the deltoid muscle should be used in older toddlers and preschoolers *(10,29–31)*. These sites have been selected for theoretical reasons, and although there is much anecdotal literature to support their appropriateness, the research literature on site selection is scant. The anterior lateral thigh was selected because it is a relatively large muscle and free of vital structures that might be injured during the injection. When the changeover should occur to the deltoid is clearly controversial. In the one article that examined this topic, Ipp and colleagues *(32)* suggested that by 18 months severe pain was identified in 30% of children injected in the thigh, but in only 8% of those injected in the arm. They also stated that 50% of children had decreased movement and ambulation when injected in the thigh at 18 months; in fact, two-thirds of that group limped for 24–48 hours following immunization. This was compared with 35% of children who had decreased arm movement when injected in the deltoid. They did report that there was more swelling and redness in the deltoid group. They suggested it is logical to change to the deltoid at 18 months based on these data.

Others disagree, however. The Los Angeles Department of Public Health *(31)* suggested that 36 months is a more appropriate time to change. The American Academy of Pediatrics *Red Book (10)* is nonspecific and suggests 18 months as the appropriate time to change sites.

Despite the limited evidence to guide practice, it is generally agreed that in young children up to 18 months, the anterior thigh (vastus lateralis) is the appropriate site for intramuscular injections, and a point between 18 and 36 months is the appropriate time to rotate to the deltoid muscle. There are unique situations in which the upper outer quadrant of the buttocks may need to be used, particularly when large volumes of injectate are necessary, such as for immune globulin. If this site is used, care must be taken to avoid injuring the sciatic nerve.

2.1.4.3. NEEDLE LENGTH

As with selection of the most appropriate site, there has been little research directed toward identifying the ideal needle length. Although it may appear intuitive that the shorter the needle is, the less pain there will be, in fact it appears that the opposite is true. Shorter needles seem to be associated with increased redness and swelling. The length of the needle chosen, however, obviously depends on the size of the child, as well as other technical variables associated with immunization technique, such as whether the skin is bunched or stretched taut. This issue is complicated by a number of contradictory studies. Diggle and Deeks *(33)* randomly assigned a sample of 4-month-old infants scheduled to receive their diphtheria–tetanus/*Haemophilis influenzae* type b vaccine in the anterolateral thigh to receive their immunization with either a 16-mm (5/8-inch) or a 25-mm (7/8-inch) needle. Over half of the infants vaccinated with the 16-mm needle developed redness and swelling initially; only one-third of the group injected with longer needle did. This distinction persisted and in fact increased by 3 days.

Two additional studies, however, called these conclusions into question. Studies by Cook and Murtagh *(34)* and Groswasser et al. *(35)* used ultrasonographic techniques to measure the subcutaneous tissue and muscle layer thickness of 2-, 4-, 6-, and 18-month-old children. Both studies identified that the shorter needle was adequate and would deposit drug in the muscle and not subcutaneous tissue if the skin was held taught and not bunched. The available data, therefore, are somewhat confusing. Zuckerman *(36)* has suggested the need for individualization of needle length based on patient size and injection technique.

In summary, it appears that in larger infants or if skin bunching is used, a longer needle is appropriate. The *Red Book* suggests needle length of 7/8 to 1 inch for infants, toddlers, and older children and 1–2 inches for adolescents and adults. There seems to be no reason not to support this suggestion. In a related matter, it had previously been suggested that aspiration of the plunger once the needle has been inserted into the muscle was important. The most recent edition of the *Red Book* suggests that the evidence for this practice is nonexistent and suggests that it is no longer necessary *(9,10)*.

2.1.4.4. Injectate Properties

In addition to the site and needle length, the properties of the injectate itself have an impact on pain. The pH of the injectate, temperature of the injectate, and type of diluent all may alter the distress associated with the immunization. Although there are very few studies that examined these factors directly for immunizations, these variables have been examined during other types of injections and may, by extrapolation, ultimately have implications for immunization pain reduction. Certainly, specific research will be necessary before any formal integration of these constructs can be endorsed.

The only studies of injectate qualities that are directly relevant at present are those that have looked at pain associated with the measles–mumps–rubella (MMR) vaccine. There have been two studies at this time *(37,38)* that have compared the traditionally administered MMR-2 vaccine with alternative immunizations (Pluserix and Priorix). Both of these vaccines appear to have a higher pH than the MMR-2. The data from Lyons and Howell *(37)* suggested that children were at least twice as likely to cry when given the MMR-2 as those given the Pluserix. Ipp and colleagues *(38)* conducted a study using VAS scores by parents, as well as videotapes of infant pain expression and pain behaviors while receiving their injections. They likewise reported a dramatic difference between the two types of immunization, with the Priorix inducing far less discomfort than the MMR-2.

Other features of the injectate may also help reduce the pain of immunization, although they have not been formally studied in this context. Based on studies of lidocaine injection, it appears that a warmer injectate causes less pain than a cold injectate *(39)*. A study by Maiden and colleagues *(40)* on temperature and immunization pain, however, called this previous work into question. They evaluated the pain of individuals over the age of 16 years who required an adult diphtheria–tetanus vaccine. The patients were randomly assigned to receive cold vaccine, rubbed vaccine (rubbed between the palms for 1 minute), or a vaccine warmed to 37°C. They found no difference in the pain scores in these groups. The role of temperature of the injectate on pain surely requires further study and may ultimately have relevance.

Another area that has not been studied for immunization pain but may also be valuable is the type of liquid used to dilute the vaccine. Because a number of these agents are not premixed (MMR, varicella, *H. influenzae* type b), it may be worthwhile to examine the use of lidocaine as a diluent instead of sterile water. It may be inferred from the work of Schichor et al. *(41)* that lidocaine may reduce injection pain when used as a diluent instead of sterile water. Their group compared the use of sterile water with lidocaine as a diluent for ceftriaxone injection and found dramatic differences initially, at 4 hours, and at 24 hours in the associated discomfort. Amir and coworkers *(42)* reported similar results when using lidocaine as a diluent for benzinathine penicillin.

2.1.5. During the Immunization

A number of strategies can be used during the injection itself that may have an impact on the pain that it produces. These include parental demeanor during the injection, the use of nonpharmacological strategies, such as distraction, as well as the use of physical strategies, such as pressure and sucrose.

2.1.5.1. Parental Demeanor

The role of parental attitude and demeanor has emerged as a critical factor in the reaction of children to immunizations. Although it seems somewhat anti-intuitive, excessive reassurance in which parents beg, plead, negotiate, or seem to apologize for the immunization is far more likely to cause distress than a more neutral response *(43,44)*. Children appeared to identify parental ambivalence toward the injection in that response pattern, and this may fuel in them an increased distress response with the hope that it can somehow cancel the immunization. It appears that a more appropriate role for parents is that of "coach" *(45)*. In that capacity, they can help their child by using distraction and other strategies that promote relaxation and active coping as compared with expressions of reassurance and sympathy, which are passive in nature and do not help with mastery.

2.1.5.2. DISTRACTION AND BREATHING

Depending on the child's age, a number of techniques are available to help relax and distract the child. In infancy, distraction may consist primarily of stroking, soothing, and softly talking to the child. In older children, however, a number of more formal strategies have been identified as effective, starting in children as young as 3 years *(46–49)*. Breathing techniques include deep breathing, blowing away shot pain through the use of pinwheels, party blowers, or bubble solution, and snake breathing (a hissing sound). Distraction techniques that have been examined include reading a favorite book to the child, listening to music, telling familiar stories, or using visual imagery to describe a favorite place and involving the child in that description *(50–52)*. Hypnosis is the more active involvement of the child in a fantasy and involves reframing the experience. These techniques are described extensively in many review articles *(53–55)*, but it is quite clear that these behavioral/cognitive techniques are well supported by evidence-based research. Factors that promote the successful use of these techniques include their developmental appropriateness for the child, matching the technique with the unique attributes and personality of the specific child, and the child's willingness to practice them at times other than immediately preceding the immunization.

2.1.5.3. LOCAL ANESTHETICS

A number of local anesthetic agents have been used during immunizations *(56–58)*. Although the depth of anesthesia that they provide varies from quite superficial for some of the refrigerant sprays to 8–9 mm for iontophoretic lidocaine, they all have a benefit of at least reducing the pain of needle insertion. Some of these agents also reduce pain subsequent to the injection itself. Eutetic mixture of local anesthetics (EMLA), amethocaine, and vapocoolant sprays have been studied specifically for reduction of injection pain. EMLA has been shown to reduce pain during the injection itself and up to 24 hours after the intramuscular injection. Both amethocaine and vapocoolant sprays have efficacy during the injection but have not been studied over the subsequent 24 hours.

There are at present a number of local anesthetic delivery systems in development (iontophoretic, heat-, and pressure-assisted delivery) that expedite the onset of anesthesia and may be more practical in the busy ambulatory setting. In general, it does appear that both refrigerant sprays and other topical agents (amethocaine, lidocaine) help somewhat with the immediate pain of injection, but refrigerant sprays may not have the prolonged analgesic benefit of the other agents.

Each practice, based on time and financial constraints, will decide on the routine use of local anesthetics for intramuscular injections. Clearly, however, for children who have developed needle phobia, the use of these agents coupled with behavioral/cognitive strategies is indicated. For other children, this remains an area of ongoing debate and evolution.

2.1.5.4. SUCROSE

Although sucrose or other sweetened liquids have been used empirically in infants to reduce the pain of procedures (e.g., a sip of wine following ritual newborn circumcision), it has only been relatively recently that this area has been formally studied. In articles by Blass and Hoffmeyer *(59)* and Barr et al. *(60)*, sucrose reduced pain associated with medical procedures (heel prick, venipuncture, circumcision) in newborns. This effect has been demonstrated in newborn infants and remains in effect for infants as old as 6 months. Sucrose has essentially no efficacy in infants older than 6 months. Investigators *(61)* have determined that, at least in part, sucrose reduces pain through stimulation of opioid receptors much as the administration of an opioid antagonist, such as naloxone appears to reverse its efficacy. Traditionally, a 24% solution of sucrose has been used, but other agents (glucose) and other concentrations have been successfully used as well.

2.1.5.5. SITE PRESSURE

Pressure at the site of injection is another strategy that has been used empirically. This concept is at least somewhat explained by the gate control theory of pain, which posits that by flooding a painful area with a non-noxious stimulus, the intensity of the painful stimulus will be reduced. Barnhill and colleagues *(62)*, in an article on adults scheduled to receive an injection, reported that those who received 10 seconds of direct pressure at the site just prior to the injection experienced a modest but statistically significant reduction in pain compared with those who did not receive site pressure. This work was replicated by Chung et al. *(63)*.

Using that basic principle, a device known as the ShotBlocker was developed. This device is a horseshoe-shaped plastic sheet with tufts on one side. It is used to provide pressure around the injection site. There are a number of unpublished studies that support its efficacy (Guevarra AD; and Gundrum T, Sherman C, and Ruhlman S, unpublished data), some with school-aged children and with adults, although some are unpublished, and their methodologies are significantly flawed.

2.1.5.6. TECHNIQUE DURING THE INJECTION

As with other aspects of immunization pain, there has been extremely limited research on the technique used to administer the injection. In general, it appears that a fast, darting motion at an angle of 90° is endorsed by most authorities for intramuscular injection. A 45° angle is appropriate for subcutaneous injection.

Likewise, there is limited literature on how a child should be restrained, in what position the child should be held, and who should do the holding during the injection. In general, young infants should be held so that a thigh is exposed, and if at all possible, the child should be positioned so the muscles relax. Often, this involves having the parent hold the child in his or her lap. Older children can either sit in the parent's lap facing the parent and with their legs wrapped around the parent (the so-called big hug) or can sit forward-facing. Either way, the deltoid should be exposed, and the muscle should be relaxed. Some parents are unable or unwilling to be involved in restraining their child, and if personnel allows, this preference should be respected.

In these days of multiple injections, there has been a debate about whether multiple immunizations should be given simultaneously or sequentially, one following the other. There have been two studies that have examined this question: one in infants and one in older children *(64,65)*. Both of these studies essentially came to the same conclusion: there is no obvious decrease in discomfort in the child if the immunizations are given simultaneously as compared to sequentially, although maximal heart rate did increase in sequential administration in infants. In both studies, however, parents seemed to prefer simultaneous administration if at all possible.

2.1.5.7. SUMMARY

Despite the frequency of intramuscular injections in children, there is a striking lack of research to support strategies aimed at pain reduction. In general, it does appear that advance preparation has some value as does the active involvement of the parents as distraction coaches. Distraction techniques should be geared toward the individual child's development and personality. An appropriate needle length and site should be used. Local anesthetics should be used based on practice logistics and previous reactions of the child to immunization. In general, sucrose should be used for infants; for in toddlers, preschoolers, and school-aged children, distraction techniques and pressure are appropriate.

2.2. Pain Associated With Common Infections

2.2.1. Otitis Media

Otitis media is the most frequent illness diagnosis made in pediatric practice for children younger than 15 years old. By 1 year, 60% of children will have been diagnosed with otitis media, and by 3 years of age, 80% of children will have had at least one episode *(66)*. In a survey by the Centers for Disease Control and Prevention in 1990, otitis media was the primary diagnosis at

24.5 million visits to the doctor *(67)*. Paradise et al. examined the records of more than 2200 Pittsburgh area infants and found antimicrobial therapy for otitis media was prescribed on average for 41 days of the first year and 48 days of the second year *(68)*.

Despite the frequency with which otitis media is diagnosed and the vast amount of antibiotics prescribed for it, there is a striking lack of data on the extent of pain associated with otitis media and the appropriate treatment of that pain. Otalgia is a frequent presenting symptom associated with otitis media. There are many pain-sensitive structures in the ear, such as the tympanic membrane, the periosteum, and the mucoperiosteum. It is logical to assume that perturbations of the ear would result in discomfort.

The role of antibiotics in the treatment of otitis remains an area of significant controversy, as does their impact on pain. Despite an increasing wealth of data, the interpretation of that information remains variable. It appears that, in randomized clinical trials, approx 60% of children with otitis media treated with either antibiotics or placebo were pain free at about 24 hours. Between 2 and 7 days after presentation, 14% of the placebo group continued to have pain; only 6% of the antibiotic group had pain. Although this difference is statistically significant and represented a 41% improvement in that antibiotic group, its clinical relevance is questionable *(69)*. To prevent 1 child from experiencing pain at 2–7 days after otitis has been diagnosed, 17 children must be treated with antibiotics. Therefore, although the impact of antibiotics may not be dramatic, they do appear to have at least a modest impact on the pain associated with otitis media. In an exchange of letters in response to an article by Damoiseaux *(70)* on antibiotics and otitis media in the *British Medical Journal*, many respondents suggested that although antibiotics may have a minor role in pain reduction, local analgesia and systemic pain relief were at least as helpful, and research was required to identify how their use could be optimized *(71)*.

There have been very few studies looking specifically at analgesic use in otitis media. Bertin et al. *(72)*, in the only randomized, double-blind, placebo-controlled trial of analgesic usage in otitis media, reported that for dosing at three times daily, pain persisted in 7% of the children with ibuprofen, 10% with acetaminophen, and 25% with placebo. Although not statistically significant, their data implies that nonsteroidal anti-inflammatory agents are probably more effective than acetaminophen for this common pain problem. Fixed preparations of acetaminophen and opioids, such as codeine, are often recommended for more pronounced pain in otitis media, although their use has never been formally studied. Hauswald and Anison *(73)*, however, in an interesting study of emergency room physicians, reported that they were more likely to prescribe narcotic analgesics for adults with severe pain associated with otitis media that prevented them from sleeping than they were for children with the same clinical picture. This study suggests the continued bias toward undertreatment of pain in children compared with adults.

It has long been known that local treatment of ear pain has benefits. Warm compresses to the ear and warmed olive oil instilled in the ear have also been used for many years. A number of articles have looked more formally at these approaches. Sarrell and coworkers *(74)* looked at advocacy of naturopathic extracts in the management of ear pain associated with acute otitis media. They found a naturopathic herbal extract reduced ear pain at least similarly to an anesthetic ear drop group. Another local treatment, Auralgan, a mixture of antipyrine, benzocaine and oxyquinolone, and glycerin, has also been shown to be effective 30 minutes following instillation *(75)*.

The area of pain management in otitis media remains controversial. There is still ongoing debate about whether antibiotics should be prescribed, although at best their impact on pain reduction is only modest. If prescribed, they should be prescribed simultaneously with analgesics, primarily a nonsteroidal anti-inflammatory drug (NSAID), such as ibuprofen. Consideration of some type of local treatment should also be entertained.

2.2.2. Pharyngitis

Acute pharyngitis is another common cause of physician office visits for children as well as adults. Pain associated with pharyngitis is variable. Of pharyngitis in children, 15–30% is secondary to group A streptococcus, and it does appear that this etiology is associated with significant pain *(76)*. In a study of all causes of pharyngitis, 80% of individuals with streptococcal pharyngitis rated their pain at least 4 out of 5, whereas those with throat pain that was nonstreptococcal in origin reported significantly less pain *(77)*.

Despite this level of discomfort, major clinical reviews of acute pharyngitis often ignore the substantial pain associated with it. In fact, Sagarin and Roberts *(78)* responded to a primary care review of acute pharyngitis in the *New England Journal of Medicine (79)* with their concern over the limited importance assigned to the assessment and management of the pain, usually the presenting symptom, in that review article. They stated that patients with pharyngitis typically come to the physician for relief of pain associated with swallowing, yet clinicians typically ignore the main reason why they have sought treatment and prescribe antibiotics, which will be of little immediate help and essentially no help if the pharyngitis is nonbacterial in origin.

For the most part, pharyngitis is a self-limited condition. After 1 week, 90% of individuals will be well, whether or not antibiotics were prescribed regardless of the origin of the pharyngitis *(80)*. It does appear, however, that for individuals with proven group A streptococcal pharyngitis, the period of pain that they experience is reduced with appropriate antibiotic therapy. For patients who have a sore throat without evidence of streptococcal pharyngitis, antibiotics have minimal effect on pain reduction.

There has been extremely limited research on the use of analgesics in pharyngitis. In one study *(77)*, ibuprofen was compared with acetaminophen and placebo. At 48 hours, pain had resolved in 80% of the patients who were on around-the-clock ibuprofen, 70% of the patients on around-the-clock acetaminophen, and 55% of patients who took placebo. Acetylsalicylic acid (or aspirin) has also been widely used for pain treatment in this condition for more than 100 years. In a double-blinded, placebo-controlled study by Eccles et al. *(81)* in adults, treatment with aspirin was found to provide relief from sore throat pain. Moore and colleagues *(82)* compared the tolerability of ibuprofen, aspirin, and acetaminophen for 7 days in patients with mild-to-moderate pain resulting from sore throat. They found 12% incidence of side effects in the ibuprofen and acetaminophen groups and a higher percentage—almost 16%— in the aspirin group. Of course, aspirin is not appropriate for use in children because of its relationship to Reye syndrome.

A number of articles have looked at the use of steroids in addition to antibiotics for severe sore throat pain. Marvez-Valls et al. *(83)* and colleagues reported on adults who presented to the emergency room with acute exudative pharyngitis. They were given an intramuscular injection of benzathine penicillin and randomly assigned to either a placebo injection or an injection of betamethasone. Those in the betamethasone group had significantly lower pain scores at follow-up 24 and 48 hours after the visit. In a similar study by Bulloch and coworkers *(84)* looked at children 5–16 years old who presented with acute pharyngitis; the children were randomly assigned to either oral dexamethasone or a placebo for pain control. In the group of children in this study who had antigen-positive streptococcal pharyngitis, the median time to clinically significant pain relief was 6 hours in the dexamethasone group vs 11 hours in the placebo group. Complete pain relief occurred at essentially the same time, about 40 hours for both groups. They suggested that the use of dexamethasone offers only limited benefit for this population.

There are a host of local treatments that have been used to improve the pain associated with pharyngitis. These include a number of local anesthetic sprays, lozenges, and gargles. At present, none of these have been rigorously investigated.

In summary, it appears that antibiotic prescription may decrease pain associated with group A streptococcal pharyngitis. Analgesics are somewhat effective as well, with ibuprofen trending toward more efficacy than acetaminophen. The role of steroids remains controversial. Local anesthetic treatments certainly should be tried, although it is difficult to recommend one specific therapy over another given the lack of evidence.

2.2.3. Pain in Viral Mouth Infections

Herpetic gingivostomatitis and herpangina are relatively common viral infections that affect infants and young children. They both cause mouth ulcers associated with significant discomfort and lead to anorexia and dehydration because of the child's unwillingness to eat or drink.

Herpetic gingivostomatitis presents with lesions on the gingiva and palate. The gingiva are red and edematous and have yellow vesicles that are often surrounded by a red halo. Herpangina, which is caused by a coxsackie A virus, presents with lesions more posteriorly placed in the mouth, in the oropharynx and posterior oral cavity.

A number of systemic treatments have been attempted for these conditions. Acyclovir has been shown to shorten the duration of lesions, as well as the duration of fever in some children *(85)*. It also may decrease eating and drinking difficulties in children who have had gingivostomatitis symptoms less than 72 hours. Other systemic strategies include the use of analgesics, either ibuprofen or acetaminophen with codeine. Children should be offered only a bland diet, avoiding irritating foods that are acidic. Dehydration should be avoided. Sometimes the use of a straw, which reduces the surface contact area with the liquid, may be helpful.

A number of local strategies have been traditionally used for viral mouth ulcers. "Magic Mouthwash" has been advocated for this condition, although its support is purely anecdotal. Magic Mouthwash consists of an agent with local activity mixed in a one-to-one concentration with agents that adhere to the ulcer *(86)*, for example, diphenhydramine plus kaopectate in a one-to-one solution.

Medications designed to help heal ulcers, such as sucralfate, have also been suggested, although there is no published literature on their use for viral mouth infections *(87)*. A mixture of polyvinyl pyrrolidone plus hyaluronic acid, marketed as Gelclair®, has been developed for pain associated with chemotherapy-induced mucositis. Innocenti et al. *(88)* reported on 30 adults who had a dramatic decrease in the pain associated with mucositis (VAS scores from 8.1 to 0.63). This product or a modification of it may ultimately have efficacy for some of the childhood viral mouth infections, but it cannot be recommended at this time.

Finally, the use of a local anesthetic agent, such as viscous lidocaine 2%, has been recommended for herpetic gingivostomatitis. This compound contains 100 mg lidocaine per 5 cc. Because a toxic dose of lidocaine is 4–5 mg/kg, it is important the product not be swallowed in large amounts, especially in infants and young children. There have been reports in the literature of significant problems associated with this compound when used inappropriately *(89)*. It is to be used when children are able to "swish and spit." If used in younger children, it should be applied with an applicator directly to the lesions.

In summary, viral mouth infections remain a significant source of distress for children. Antiviral agents may provide some relief, but systemic analgesics coupled with local treatments are the mainstay of pain relief at this time.

3. Chronic Pain

There are a number of chronic pain syndromes commonly seen in pediatric offices and clinics. Chronic pain is traditionally defined as pain existing recurrently or consistently in the previous 3 months *(8)*. The American Pain Society has added to that definition that chronic pain, in contrast to acute pain, rarely is accompanied by autonomic arousal *(90)*. Chronic pain is a remarkably frequent occurrence in children and has an overall prevalence ranging between 15 and 25%. Girls tend to have more chronic pain than boys (30 vs 19%). Chronic pain in childhood seems to peak between 12 and 15 years, but it is still significant in children as late as 16–18 years *(91)*.

Typical chronic problems are headache, abdominal pain, and limb pain. Of children who report chronic pain, 50% have pain in multiple sites, and the incidence of multiple pain sites increases with age. In children who have multiple pain sites, the most common combination is headache and abdominal pain, which occurs in 25% of all cases *(92)*.

Chronic pain has a significant impact on the child who experiences it, as well as on his or her family and on the health care system. For children, there are often problems with adjustment, school performance, and social skills as they are removed or remove themselves from the social arena because of discomfort *(93)*. School performance suffers as well, and school absenteeism is frequent. In particular, children with headache, irritable bowel syndrome, and widespread musculoskeletal pain are frequently absent from school. School absenteeism places a burden on parents, who often must miss work as a result. This may have significant economic impact on the family, which further exacerbates the family stress and discord that often accompany chronic pain.

Perquin and colleagues *(94)* examined the impact of childhood chronic pain on the health care system. Of the 25% of survey respondents who reported chronic pain, 57% of that group required physician consultation, and 39% were on continuous medication. They did not address the economic impact of hospitalization, ongoing diagnostic evaluation, or other interventions for this population.

The evaluation of chronic pain often falls on the already-burdened shoulders of the office-based practitioner. The evaluation and management of these problems is often complex and time-consuming. Elaborate algorithms have been developed to address the very lengthy list of potential etiologies for these problems. Physicians often fear that, despite extensive evaluation, an organic explanation may be uncovered in the next series of investigations. It is hard as a result to draw the diagnostic "line in the sand" when it is felt that enough investigation has already occurred. Physicians will often state that "for the sake of completeness" they will continue investigating the problem even though they genuinely believe that the symptom is unlikely to have a defined organic explanation. Families perceive this continued investigation as evidence of a lurking organic explanation that is yet to be uncovered, and they press the physician for even further testing or search for another physician who will orchestrate additional and often more invasive investigation. When extensive and expensive testing does not yield a conclusive explanation, the physician will often designate the symptom as "psychosomatic" or "functional," attributions that are usually unhelpful and often inaccurate. The art of medicine in this area is identifying the red flags in the history, physical, and initial laboratory investigations that suggest that additional investigation might be warranted on the one hand while not extensively overmedicalizing the problem on the other. During this period of evaluation, which Eccleston has called a "diagnostic vacuum" *(95)*, the child's pain should be treated.

Detailed discussion of the evaluation of each of the common chronic pain problems (abdominal pain, back pain, headache, limb pain, widespread musculoskeletal pain) is significantly beyond the scope of this chapter, and there are excellent review articles available. In addition to the typical aspects of the history and physical that are considered for each of these pain problems, a few aspects of the routine evaluation that are not often discussed but may yield additional information deserve emphasis.

From the biological side, hypermobility frequently co-occurs with many types of chronic pain, especially limb, back, and widespread musculoskeletal pain *(96,97)*. Although the nature of this relationship (causation vs correlation) is not certain, using a Beighton scale *(98)* or other measure to identify hypermobility often yields positive results and may offer a hypothesis for the etiology of the child's discomfort.

All evaluation of chronic pain should include some psychological assessment. This does not imply causation, but there may be a transactional relationship between chronic pain and anxiety and depression, with pain yielding anxiety and depression and depression/anxiety exacerbating pain. Evaluating the child for these problems should not be perceived as implying a "psychogenic" explanation for the child's discomfort. It should be explained to the family that all pain, particularly chronic pain, has psychological and physiological components. Any comprehensive evaluation and any treatment plan should contain all of those elements.

Along similar lines, the child's school experience should be examined. Learning disabilities and attentional problems not infrequently complicate chronic pain. It is also imperative to discuss social factors at school and inquire about bullying. These factors should not be construed as the "cause" of the pain *per se* but may have a role in amplifying the child's interpretation of the pain signal. All pain is, of course, the composite of the nociceptive input and the interpretation of that input.

There are a number of general principles about the treatment of chronic pain as well. Again, these should be considered along with the specific strategies for the particular pain problem. Treatment should be multimodal from the outset, as almost all pain problems have biological, psychological, social, and educational components. When dealing with chronic pain, success should be measured not only by decreased pain intensity ratings, but also perhaps more importantly by improved function. This may include mood, activities of daily living, school attendance, involvement with friends, "joie de vivre," sleep, appetite, and so on. These functional markers are a more sensitive indication of improvement than self-reports of pain intensity, which may not decrease initially.

A critical aspect of treatment for all chronic pain problems is the initial explanation to the child and family. It is important to convey the message that the clinician is familiar with the symptom complex that the child has, and that it is not life threatening, even if the exact problem is not clearly defined. Most important, we help them distinguish the notion of "hurt" from the notion of "harm" *(99)*. We explain that, in chronic pain, the protective or warning function of the pain message that is the hallmark of acute pain is no longer operative.

Chronic persistent pain does not imply that progressive damage is occurring, as might be expected with acute pain (e.g., if we leave our hand on a stove or walk on a broken leg). It is critical for parents and children to understand this for a number of reasons. First, it may reduce the urgency that parents feel to identify the exact cause of the problem. Second, many of the treatment strategies used for chronic pain may in fact require the child to experience a slight increase in discomfort in the short run (physical therapy, school attendance, social interaction). Parents may be far more willing to comply with requests to encourage normal behavior if they do not feel that this will cause further deterioration.

At the outset of treatment, parents should be informed that the child will be monitored carefully through scheduled follow-up visits. It is reassuring to families and validating that, even if a potential biological explanation for the child's discomfort was not identified initially, a system of monitoring is in place to identify changes in symptoms that may imply the need for alternative investigations or treatments. This has been labeled "watchful waiting" *(100)*; obviously, if a pain problem does not evolve or change significantly over time, it strongly mitigates against an ongoing progressive disease.

Monitoring of symptoms can be aided through the use of a symptom diary. This allows the child to participate in his or her own care and alerts the clinician to new or changed symptoms. It can also be used to monitor the success of the intervention. It is important that the focus of the diary be on symptoms and function (mood, time with friends, school attendance) and not solely on pain intensity ratings, which are often unchanging.

Individuals with chronic pain often have problems sleeping *(101)*. Attention to sleep hygiene should be given, and medications should only be used when necessary. Amitriptyline, which may be effective in the treatment of neuropathic pain, has the useful side effect of sedation, which helps with sleep onset. Melatonin and trazodone may also be beneficial.

A number of other medications may be helpful, but it is important not to overmedicate children with chronic pain. Depending on the nature of the pain, NSAIDs may be used around the clock or as needed. Tramadol is often helpful for more severe pain, and tricyclic antidepressants may be beneficial in widespread pain or pain that may have a neuropathic component. Obviously, medications for specific pain problems may have value, such as NSAIDs plus caffeine for headache or famotidine or pizotifen for abdominal pain *(102)*.

Physical therapy is often the cornerstone of the treatment of chronic pain *(103)*. Interventions include general conditioning for problems like fibromyalgia, desensitization for reflex sympathetic dystrophy, and stretching or strengthening particular muscle groups. In addition, therapy such as transcutaneous electrical nerve stimulation, heat, and massage may benefit certain pain problems. There has been limited controlled research in this area, but anecdotally a graduated physical exercise program appears to be an important intervention in the treatment of many chronic and persistent pains. Whether this represents the impact of the therapy itself, the ongoing relationship with a helping, caring professional, or improvement in self-efficacy when success is achieved is unclear. Regardless, there are reasonable data to suggest that physical therapy is essential for the adequate treatment of chronic and persistent pain.

Likewise, cognitive-behavioral strategies are also valuable and are indicated for all pain problems, regardless of origin *(104,105)*. These strategies are often helpful during acute pain suffering, and there are limited data on their efficacy for chronic pain, although anecdotally they seem to be effective. Strategies include meditation, distraction, use of biofeedback, and hypnosis. They may be taught by the primary care provider, a psychologist, or another skilled individual. If possible, this should occur during relatively pain-free periods and not in the middle of severe pain episodes.

Parents have a critical role in decreasing chronic pain. They need to encourage normal behavior and deemphasize responding to pain escalations. This can be done sympathetically without appearing to ignore the pain, but by positively emphasizing the virtue of coping, parents can encourage children to practice cognitive behavioral strategies and can function as a coach emphasizing those strategies during painful episodes or procedures.

Attention to schoolwork and attendance is critical as well. In children with chronic and persistent pain, development of a modification program may be necessary. In the United States, this program is sometimes known as a 504 plan and stems from the Rehabilitation Act of 1973. The program should be tailored to the child's specific needs and may allow for alterations in the length of the schoolday as well as modifications of homework volume. Regardless of the program, school attendance should be mandatory, and if the child has not been attending school for a time, graduated reentry with supportive tutoring can be developed. In such a situation, the school nursing office can be a sanctuary and temporary refuge where the child can rest and be removed from the stress of school. It is sometimes helpful to develop a "script" for the child to use on reentry to school and to offer specific phrases to use when other children ask about his or her absence.

Specific criteria for staying home also need to be developed. Parents need to be as consistent as they possibly can in this area. For example, children should go to school every day unless they have a fever. This eliminates the inevitable parental vacillation, which is quite common in children with chronic pain. Each morning, parents must try to assess the child's level of comfort and disability when confronted with the child's report of escalating discomfort. Such a plan gives parents criteria by which they can make informed decisions regarding school attendance.

In general, the overall approach to chronic pain in the primary care setting is to evaluate the history, physical examination, and screening laboratory assessments for red flags that might suggest organic disease. Testing should be kept to a minimum unless there are specific indications for additional tests. The child and family should then be informed that no progressive illness was identified, and that the child's clinical picture is similar to many other children. Regardless, families should be reassured that the child will be carefully monitored over time. The primary care provider needs to keep a positive attitude and needs to function as a cheerleader, reinforcing any successes that the child may have. Frequent follow-up visits should be scheduled so that the family can feel comfortable that evolving organic disease will not be missed. Typical interventions include physical therapy and cognitive/behavioral strategies with medications targeted to specific symptoms. Success should be monitored by improvement in function and not specifically through reduction in pain intensity scales.

4. Conclusion

Despite its frequency, pain in the pediatric office has been grossly under-researched. It does appear that simple changes can yield a significant reduction in pain in that setting. The pain of immunizations can clearly be reduced through the selection of the appropriate site and needle, through the routine use of physical and psychological techniques, and through the use of local anesthetics. Reduction in immunization pain may increase compliance with subsequent immunizations and decrease anticipatory anxiety over future visits to the doctor.

Pain associated with common infectious diseases, such as otitis media, pharyngitis, and viral mouth infections, can be reduced with systemic and local approaches.

Chronic pains, such as headache, recurrent abdominal pain, limb pain, and widespread musculoskeletal pain, are also common symptoms presenting to the pediatric office. It is critical that they be investigated adequately to rule out pathological conditions, but not so extensively that they create the impression that there is an underlying medical cause waiting around the next laboratory bend. Treatment usually involves explaining the distinction between hurt and harm, appropriate monitoring, and a cluster of approaches that involve physical activity and cognitive behavioral strategies with analgesics for the occasional severe pain episode.

Even though all pain in ambulatory settings cannot realistically be relieved, merely acknowledging it and attempting to address it is an important first step. Introducing some of the simple strategies discussed in this chapter will go a long way to reassuring the children and families for whom we care that their comfort, as well as their health, is our concern.

Acknowledgments

The author acknowledges the generous support of the Rockfeller Foundation Bellagio Study and Conference Center, where much of this chapter was written.

References

1. Schechter NL, Berde CB, Yaster M. Pain in infants, children, and adolescents: an overview. In: Schechter NL, Berde CB, Yaster M, eds. Pain in Infants, Children, and Adolescents, 2nd ed. Philadelphia: Lippincott, Williams, and Wilkins; 2003, pp. 3–18.
2. Anand KJS, Sippell WG, Aynsley-Green A. Randomized trial of fentanyl anesthesia in preterm babies undergoing surgery: effects on stress response. Lancet 1987;1:243–248.
3. Goldschneider KR, Anand KJS. Long term consequences of pain in neonates. In: Schechter NL, Berde CB, Yaster M, eds. Pain in Infants, Children, and Adolescents, 2nd ed. Philadelphia: Lippincott, Williams, and Wilkins; 2003, pp. 58–67.
4. World Health Organization. Cancer Pain and Palliative Care in Children. Geneva: World Health Organization; 1998.
5. Ljungman G, Gordh T, Sorensen S, et al. Pain in paediatric oncology: interviews with children, adolescents, and their parents. Acta Paediatr 1999;88:623–630.

6. Tohill J, McMorrow O. Pain relief in the neonatal intensive care unit. Lancet 1996;336:569.
7. Anand KJ. International Evidence-Based Group for Neonatal Pain. Consensus statement for the prevention and management of pain in the newborn. Arch Pediatr Adolesc Med 2001;155:173–180.
8. McGrath PJ, Finley GA. Chronic and Recurrent Pain in Children and Adolescents. Progress in Pain Research and Management. Vol. 13. Seattle, WA: IASP Press; 1999.
9. Pickering LK. Red Book: 2003 Report of the Committee on Infectious Diseases. 26th ed. Elk Grove, IL: American Academy of Pediatrics; 2003.
10. Committee on Infectious Diseases, American Academy of Pediatrics. Red Book: 2003 Report of the Committee on Infectious Diseases. 26th ed. Elk Grove Village, IL: American Academy of Pediatrics; 2003.
11. Fassler D. The fear of needles in children. Am J Orthopsychiatry 1985;55:371–377.
12. Menke E. School-aged children's perception of stress in the hospital. Child Health Care 1981;9:80–86.
13. Ornstein P, Manning EL, Pelphrey KA. Children's memory for pain. J Dev Behav Pediatr 1999;20:262–277.
14. Taddio A, Katz J, Ilersich AL. Effect of neonatal circumcision on pain response during subsequent routine vaccination. Lancet 1997;349:599–603.
15. Fitzgerald M, Millard C, McIntosh N. Cutaneous hypersensitivity following peripheral tissue damage in newborn infants and its reversal with topical anaesthesia. Pain 1989;39:31.
16. Weisman SJ, Bernstein B, Schechter NL. Consequences of inadequate analgesia during painful procedures in children. Arch Pediatr Adolesc Med 1998;152: 147–149.
17. Schechter NL, Bernstein BA, Beck A, et al. Individual differences in children's response to pain: role of temperament and parental characteristics. Pediatrics 1991;87:171–177.
18. Beyer JE, Villarruel AM, Denyes MJ. The Oucher: User's Manual and Technical Report. Bethesda, MD: Association for the Care of Children's Health; 1995.
19. Katz ER, Kellerman J, Siegel SE. Distress behavior in children with cancer undergoing medical procedures: developmental considerations. J Consult Clin Psychol 1980;48:356–365.
20. Chen E, Craske MG, Katz ER, Schwartz E, Zeltzer LK. Pain-sensitive temperament: does it predict procedural distress and response to psychological treatment among children with cancer? J Pediatr Psychol 2000;25:269–278.
21. Lee LW, White-Traut RC. The role of temperament in pediatric pain response. Issues Compr Pediatr Nurs 1996;19:49–63.
22. Meyerhoff AS, Weniger BG, Jacobs J. Economic value to parents of reducing the pain and emotional distress of childhood vaccine injections. Pediatr Infect Dis 2001;20:s57–s62.
23. Reis EC, Jacobson RM, Tarbell S, et al. Taking the sting out of shots: control of vaccination-associated pain and adverse reactions. Pediatr Ann 1998;27:375–386.

24. Singer T, Seymour B, O'Doherty J, Kaube H, Dolan RJ, Frith CD. Empathy for pain involves the affective but not sensory components of pain. Science 2004;303:1157–1162.
25. Woodin KA, Rodewald LE, Humiston SG, et al. Are children becoming pincushions from immunizations? Arch Pediatr Adolesc Med 1995;149:845–849.
26. Reis EC. Multiple scheduled injections contribute to missed opportunities to immunize during well care visits [abstract]. Ambul Child Health 1997;3(1, pt 2):172.
27. Fernald CD, Corry JJ. Empathic vs directive preparation of children for needles. Child Health Care 1981;10:44–46.
28. Zeltzer L, Jay SM, Fisher DM. The management of pain associated with pediatric procedures. Pediatr Clin North Am 1989;36:941–964.
29. Royal College of Paediatrics and Child Health. Position Statement on Injection Technique. London Royal College of Paediatrics and Child Health, 2002.
30. World Health Organization. Expanded Programme on Immunization. Geneva: World Health Organization; 1998.
31. County of Los Angeles Department of Public Health. Immunizations: minimizing pain and maximizing comfort. Public Health 2001;1:3.
32. Ipp MM, Gold R, Goldebach M, et al. Adverse reactions to diphtheria, tetanus, pertussis-polio vaccination at 18 mo of age: effect of injection site and needle length. Pediatrics 1989;83:670–682.
33. Diggle L, Deeks J. Effect of needle length on incidence of local reactions to routine immunization in infants aged 4 mo: randomized controlled trial. BMJ 2000;321:931–933.
34. Cook IF, Murtagh J. Needle length required for intramuscular vaccination of infants and toddlers. Aust Fam Physician 2002;31:295–297.
35. Groswasser J, Kahn A, Bouche B, et al. Needle length and injection technique for efficient intramuscular vaccine delivery in infants and children evaluated through an ultrasonographic determination of subcutaneous and muscle layer thickness. Pediatrics 1997;100:400–403.
36. Zuckerman JN. The importance of injecting vaccines into muscle: different patients need different needle sizes. BMJ 2000;321:1237, 1238.
37. Lyons R, Howell F. Pain and measles, mumps, and rubella vaccination. Arch Dis Child 1991;66:346–367.
38. Ipp M, Cohen E, Goldbach M, Macarthur C. Effect of choice of measles-mumps-rubella vaccine on immediate vaccination pain in infants. Arch Pediatr Adolesc Med 2004;158:323–326.
39. Bartfield JM, Crisafulli KM, Raccio-Robak N, Salluzzo RF. The effects of warming and buffering on pain of infiltration of lidocaine. Acad Emerg Med 1995; 2:254–257.
40. Maiden MJ, Benton GN, Bourne RA. Effect of warming adult diphtheria-tetanus vaccine on discomfort after injection: a randomized controlled trial. Med J Aust 2003;178:433–436.
41. Schichor A, Bernstein B, Weinerman H, et al. Lidocaine as a diluent for ceftriaxone in the treatment of gonorrhea: does it reduce the pain of injection? Arch Dis Pediatr Adolesc Med 1994;148:72–75.

42. Amir J, Ginat S, Cohen YH et al. Lidocaine as a diluent for the administration of benzathine penicillin G. Pediatr Infect Dis J 1998;17:890–893.
43. Blount RL, Bachanas P, Powers S, et al. Training children to cope and parents to coach them during routine immunizations: effects on child, parent, and staff behaviors. Behav Ther 1992;23:689–705.
44. Cohen LL, Manimala MR, Blount RL. Easier said than done: what parents say they do and what they do during child's immunizations. Child Health Care 2000; 29:79–86.
45. Manimala MR, Blount RL, Cohen LL. The effects of parental reassurance vs distraction on child distress during immunizations. Child Health Care 2000;229: 161–177.
46. Manne SL, Redd WH, Jacobsen PB, et al. Behavioral intervention to reduce child and parent distress during venipuncture. J Consult Clin Psychol 1994;58:556–566.
47. French FM, Painter EC, Coury DL. Blowing away shot pain: a technique for pain management during immunization. Pediatrics 1994;93:384–388.
48. Fowler Kerry S, Lander J. Management of injection pain in children. Pain 1987; 30:169–175.
49. Sparks L. Taking the "ouch" out of injections for children: using distraction to decrease pain. Am J Matern Child Nurs 2001;26:72–78.
50. Cohen LL. Reducing infant immunization distress through distraction. Health Psychol 2002;21:207–211.
51. Kuttner L. Management of young children's acute pain and anxiety during invasive medical procedures. Pediatrician 1989;16:39–44.
52. Zeltzer L, LeBaron S. Hypnotic and nonhypnotic techniques for reduction of pain and anxiety during painful procedures in children and adolescents with cancer. J Pediatr 1982;101:1032–1035.
53. Ellis JA, Spanos NP. Cognitive-behavioral interventions for children's distress during bone marrow aspirations and lumbar punctures: a critical review. J Pain Symptom Manage 1994;9:96–108.
54. Chen E, Joseph MH, Zeltzer LK. Behavioral and cognitive interventions in the treatment of pain in children. Pediatr Clin North Am 2000;47:513–525.
55. Kazak AE, Penati B, Brophy P, Himelstein B. Pharmacologic and psychologic interventions for procedural pain. Pediatrics 1998;102(1, pt 1):59–66.
56. Halperin DL, Koren G, Attias D, et al. Topical skin anesthesia for venous, subcutaneous drug reservoir and lumbar punctures in children. Pediatrics 1989;84: 281–284.
57. Reis EC, Holobukov R. Vapoocoolant spray is equally effective as EMLA cream in reducing immunization pain in school-aged children. Pediatrics 1997;100: e1025–e1029.
58. O'Brien L, Taddio A, Ipp M, et al. Topical 4% amethocaine gel reduces the pain of subcutaneous measles-mumps-rubella vaccination. Pediatrics 2004;114:6: e720–e724.
59. Blass E, Hoffmeyer LB. Sucrose as an analgesic for newborn infants. Pediatrics 1991;87:215–218.

60. Barr RG, Young SN, Wright JH, et al. "Sucrose analgesia" and diphtheria-tetanus-pertussis immunizations at 2 and 4 mo. J Dev Behav Pediatr 1995;16:220–225.

61. Blass EM, Cramer CP, Fanselow MS. The development of morphine-induced antinociception in neonata rats: a comparison of forepaw, hindpaw, and tail retraction from a thermal stimulus. Pharmacol Biochem Behav 1993;44:643–649.

62. Barnhill BJ, Holbert MD, Jackson NM, Erickson RS. Using pressure to decrease the pain of intramuscular injections. J Pain Symptom Manage 1996;12:52–58.

63. Chung JWY, Ng WMY, Wong TKS. An experimental study on the use of manual pressure to reduce pain in intramuscular injections. J Clin Nurs 2002;11:457–461.

64. Horn MI, McCArthy AM. Children's responses to sequential vs simultaneous immunization injections. J Pediatr Health Care 1999;13:18–23.

65. Bogin FJ, Bernstein BA, Payton JS, Schechter NL, Ristau B. A comparison of the pain associated with simultaneous (SIM) vs sequential (SEQ) immunization injection given at the 9 and 12 mo well child visits. Pediatr Res 2004;55:210A.

66. Rosenfeld R, Bluestone C. Evidence-based otitis media. St. Louis, MO: Decker; 1999.

67. Schappert SM. Office Visits for Otitis Media: United States, 1975–2000. Hyattsville, MD: National Center for Health Statistics; 1–18. Data from Vital and Health Statistics of the Centers for Disease Control No. 214, 2003.

68. Paradise JL, Rockette JE, Colborn K, et al. Otitis media in 2253 Pittsburgh area infants: prevalence and risk factors during the first 2 yr of life. Pediatrics 1997;99:318–333.

69. Del Mar C, Glaszious P, Hayem M. Are antibiotics indicated as initial treatment for children with acute otitis media: a meta analysis. BMJ 1997;314:1526–1529.

70. Damoiseaux RAMJ, van Balen FAM, Hoes AW, et al. Primary care based randomised double blind trial of amoxicillin vs placebo for acute otitis media in children under 2 yr. BMJ 2000;320:350–354.

71. Cantekin EI. Time to stop misuse of antibiotics [letter]. BMJ 2000;321:765.

72. Bertin L, Pons G, D'Athis P, et al. A randomized, double-blind, multicentre controlled trial of ibuprofen vs acetaminophen and placebo for symptoms of acute otitis media in children. Fundam Clin Pharmacol 1996;10:378–392.

73. Hauswald M, Anison C. Prescribing analgesics: the effect of patient age and physician specialty. Pediatr Emerg Care 1997;13:262, 263.

74. Sarrell EM, Mandelberg A, Cohen HA. Efficacy of naturopathic extracts in the management of ear pain associated with acute otitis media. Arch Pediatr Adolesc Med 2001;155:796–799.

75. Hoberman A, Paradise JL, Reynolds EA, et al. Efficacy of Auralgan for treating ear pain in children with acute otitis media. Arch Pediatr Adolesc Med 1997; 151:675–678.

76. Poses RM, Cebul RD, Collins M, et al. The accuracy of experienced physicians' estimates for patients with sore throats: implications for decision-making. JAMA 1985;254:925–929.

77. Bertin L, Pons G, d'Athis P, et al. Randomized double-blind multi-center, controlled trial of ibuprofen vs acetaminophen for symptoms of tonsillitis and pharyngitis in children. J Pediatr 1991;119:811–814.

78. Sagarin MJ, Roberts J. Acute Pharyngitis [correspondence]. N Engl J Med 2001;344:1479–1480.
79. Bisno AL. Primary care: acute pharyngitis. N Engl J Med 2001;344:205–211.
80. Del Mar C, Glasziou P. Antibiotics for the symptoms and complications of sore throat. In: Cochrane Collaboration. Cochrane Library. Issue 3. Oxford, UK: Update Software; 1998.
81. Eccles R, Loose I, Jawad M, et al. Effects of acetylsalicylic acid on sore throat pain and other pain symptoms associated with acute upper respiratory infection. Pain Med 2003;4:118–124.
82. Moore N, LeParc JM, van Ganse E, et al. Tolerability of ibuprofen, aspirin and paracetamol for the treatment of cold and flu symptoms and sore throat pain. Int J Clin Pract 2002;56:732–734.
83. Marvez-Valls EG, Ernst AA, Gray J, Johnson WD. The role of betamethasone in the treatment of excudative pharyngitis. Acad Emerg Med 1998;5:567–572.
84. Bulloch B, Kabani, Tenenbein M. Oral dexamethasone for the treatment of pain in children with acute pharyngitis. Ann Emerg Med 2003;41:601–608.
85. Amir J, Harel L, Smetana Z. Treatment of herpes simplex gingivostomatitis with acyclovir in children. BMJ 1997;314:1800–1803.
86. Peter JR, Haney HM. Infections of the oral cavity. Pediatr Ann 1996;25:573.
87. Freeman SB, Markwell JK. Sucralfate in alleviating post-tonsillectomy pain. Laryngoscope 1992;102:1242–1246.
88. Innocenti M, Moscatelli G, Lopez S. Efficacy of Gelclair in reducing pain in palliative care patients with oral lesions: preliminary findings from an open pilot study. J Pain Symptom Manage 2002;24:456–457.
89. Gonzalez del Rey J, Wason S, Druckenbrod RW. Lidocaine overdose: another preventable case? Pediatr Emerg Care 1994;10:344–346.
90. American Pain Society. Principles of Analgesic Use in the Treatment of Acute and Cancer Pain. 4th ed. Glenview, IL: American Pain Society; 1999, p. 4.
91. Goodman JE, McGrath PJ. The epidemiology of pain in children and adolescents: a review. Pain 1991;46:247–264.
92. Kristjansdottir G. Prevalence of pain combinations and overall pain: a study of headache, stomach pain and back pain among schoolchildren. Scan J Soc Med 1997;25:58–63.
93. Palmero TM. Impact of recurrent and chronic pain on child and family daily functioning: a critical review of the literature. J Dev Behav Pediatr 2000;21:58–69.
94. Perquin CW, Hazebrpel-Kampschreur AA, Hunfeld JA, et al. Pain in children and adolescents: a common problem. Pain 2000;87:51–58.
95. Eccleston C, Malleson P. Managing chronic pain in children and adolescents. BMJ 2003;326:1408–1409.
96. Engelbert RH, Bank RA, Sakkers RJ, Helders PJ, Beemer FA, Uiterwaal CS. Pediatric generalized joint hypermobility with and without musculoskeletal complaints: a localized or systemic disorder? Pediatrics 2003;111:e248–e254.
97. Barron DF, Cohen BA, Geraghty MT, Violand R, Rowe PC. Joint hypermobility is more common in children with chronic fatigue syndrome than in healthy controls. J Pediatr 2002;141:421–425.

98. Grahame R. The revised (Beighton 1998) criteria for the diagnosis of benign joint hypermobility syndrome. J Rheumatol 2000;27:1777–1779.

99. Walco GA, Cassidy RC, Schechter NL. Pain, hurt, and harm. The ethics of pain control in infants and children. N Engl J Med 1994;331:541–544.

100. Herzog DB, Harper G. Unexplained disability: diagnostic dilemmas and principles of management. Clin Pediatr 1981;20:761–768.

101. Lewin DS, Dahl RE. Importance of sleep in the management of pediatric pain. J Dev Behav Pediatr 1999;20:244–252.

102. Weydert JA, Ball TM, Davis MF. Systematic review of treatments for recurrent abdominal pain. Pediatrics 2003;111:e1.

103. Sherry DD, Wallace CA, Kelley C, Kidder M, Sapp L. Short- and long-term outcomes of children with complex regional pain syndrome type I treated with exercise therapy. Clin J Pain 1999;15:218–223.

104. Eccleston C, Yorke L, Morley S, et al. Psychological therapies for the management of chronic and recurrent pain in children and adolescents. Cochrane Database of Systematic Reviews 2004.

105. Walco GA, Sterling CM, Conte PM, Engel RG. Empirically supported treatments in pediatric psychology: disease-related pain. J Pediatr Psychol 1999;24:155–167.

3

Pain and Pain Relief in Pediatric End-of-Life Care

John J. Collins and Gerri Frager

Summary

The pain experienced at the end of a child's life is a complexity of physical, psycho-logical, social, spiritual, and other factors. All factors in this matrix must be considered and treated to effect a successful system of care for a dying child. It is only in recent years that the special needs of the dying child and the child's family have been recognized and spe-cialized pediatric palliative care services developed. There is a small but evolving collec-tive expertise that is developing clinical services to care for dying children. The knowledge base also is small but evolving. The collective knowledge base will grow more quickly with time if this endeavor becomes an international collaborative effort.

Key Words: Child; dying; end of life; evidence; life limiting; pain; palliative care; pediatric; symptoms.

1. Introduction

Pain and pain relief in pediatric end-of-life care is a complex matrix caused and exacerbated potentially by a multitude of factors, including physical, psychological, social, spiritual, and other issues. All factors in this matrix must be considered and treated to effect a successful system of care. Pediatric pallia-tive care is best delivered by a multidisciplinary team involved in the care of children with life-limiting illnesses. Palliative care may begin at diagnosis, and for children with slowly progressive illnesses, palliative care may last for years. A common misconception, based on an older, traditional model, erroneously equates palliative care with terminal care. This discussion focuses primarily on the end-of-life component within the broader context of palliative care.

It is only in recent years that the special needs of the dying child and the child's family have been recognized and specialized pediatric palliative care services developed. One impelling force in this development has been the World Health Organization document *Cancer Pain Relief and Palliative Care*

From: *Bringing Pain Relief to Children: Treatment Approaches*
Edited by: G. A. Finley, P. J. McGrath, and C. T. Chambers © Humana Press Inc., Totowa, NJ

in Children (1), which raised the expectation, irrespective of geographical location, that every child with cancer should be offered a minimum standard of pain relief and palliative care. Although written with the child having cancer in mind, the principles are applicable to any child living with or dying with a condition requiring their pain and palliative care needs addressed. The document, although acknowledging that treatment options for some children are limited, expects that pain relief and palliative care should be part of the standard of care offered to every child. Apart from the humanitarian perspective to alleviate suffering in our fellow human being, another driving force toward a better standard of pain management in dying children is the insight that their unrelieved pain and suffering will be carried for many years in the memories of their parents *(2)*.

2. End-of-Life Care in Children: The Magnitude of the Problem

Globally, 12.2 million children younger than 5 years die each year *(3)*, and many of these children have life-limiting illnesses for which palliative care could be beneficial *(3)*. The causes of mortality differ vastly depending on geographical location and the availability of treatment options. Sadly, in many countries, treatment options for cancer and HIV/AIDS are limited, and palliative care as the sole focus may increase earlier in a given disease trajectory.

The data regarding pain and other symptoms experienced by children at the end of life are often from retrospective chart reviews. These data conform to the following three categories: general symptom data on children at the end of life, disease-specific data on pain and other symptoms experienced at the end of life, and general symptom data in the context of life-limiting illness.

2.1. General Symptom Data on Children at the End of Life

2.1.1. Pain and Other Symptoms at the End of a Child's Life

A retrospective chart review examined the signs and symptoms occurring at the end of life in 28 children dying from cancer in Japan. All children experienced anorexia, 82.1% had dyspnea, and 75% had pain. Other symptoms included fatigue (71.4%), nausea/vomiting (57.1%), constipation (46.4%), and diarrhea (21.4%) *(4)*. This symptom profile parallels that of the North American reviews of the symptoms of dying children *(2,5,6)*.

The proxy report of nurses caring for children during their last days of life, the majority (66.7%) of whom died in the intensive care unit, documented their symptoms with a modified Memorial Symptom Assessment Scale *(7,8)*. A mean of 11.1 ± 5.6 symptoms were documented per child. At least half of the children had six symptoms, with the most frequent being lack of energy, drowsiness, skin changes, irritability, pain, and extremity swelling. Lack of energy was the most distressing symptom for nearly one-third of the children. Nervousness, worry, and dysesthetic extremities were notably distressing, although not frequent.

The majority of children were described in the health professionals' notes as "always comfortable" to "usually comfortable" in the last week (64%), day (76.6%), and hour (93.4%) of life.

2.2. Disease-Specific Data on Pain and Other Symptoms at End of Life

2.2.1. Pain in Children With Cystic Fibrosis at the End of Life

A retrospective chart review at a tertiary care hospital was conducted summarizing the end-of-life care of US patients more than 5 years old dying from cystic fibrosis *(9)*. Of these patients, 25% had been receiving opioids for the treatment of chronic headache or chest pain for more than their last 3 months of life. When opioids were used for the treatment of breathlessness or chest pain, the proportion increased to 86%. When pain was present, it was described as "serious" pain, with chest, head, extremity, abdomen, and back the more common locations *(10)*. Increasing pain for this patient population may signal advanced progressive disease *(10)*.

2.3. General Symptom Data in the Context of Life-Limiting Illness

2.3.1. Pain in Children With Cancer

The pattern of symptoms based on the self-report of US children aged 10–18 years treated for cancer was studied *(7)*. This study included children across the spectrum of illness and included newly diagnosed patients, those receiving a bone marrow transplant, and those receiving palliative care. It showed that children with cancer are very symptomatic and are often highly distressed by their symptoms. A prevalence rate greater than 35% was noted for the symptoms of pain, drowsiness, nausea, cough, anorexia, lack of energy, and psychological upset. Inpatients reported being more symptomatic than their outpatient cohort, as evidenced by comparing their mean number of symptoms of 12.7 ± 4.9 and 6.5 ± 5.7, respectively.

Recent administration of chemotherapy is associated with significant symptomatology in children with cancer *(7)*. Children with solid tumors were more symptomatic than children with other malignancies. Pain, nausea, and anorexia were clustered as highly distressing symptoms *(7)*. Children 7–12 years old, also treated for cancer, similarly self-reported their symptoms over a 2-day period. In the realm of physical symptoms, the most prevalent, many of which were reported as highly distressing, were pain, difficulty sleeping, itch, nausea, fatigue, and anorexia *(11)*.

2.3.2. Pain and Other Symptoms in Children With Neurodegenerative Illnesses

Pain, breathlessness, and oral symptoms (i.e., secretions) were highlighted as the most common symptoms by caregiver's proxy report for children in the last month of life at an inpatient hospice *(12)*. Half of the children in the study were noncommunicative, with neurodegenerative illness a prominent diagnosis in this patient population.

JAKE'S STORY: A CASE REPORT OF A CHILD WITH NEUROCOGNITIVE IMPAIRMENT

Jake is a 10-month-old with marked irritability and apparent pain-related behaviors associated with a progressive neurodegenerative disorder resulting from an inborn error of metabolism expected to result in his death within the next 1–2 years. In addition to lack of extremity use for purposeful movement, spasticity and hypertonicity are prominent features of his condition. Jake was empirically started on a scheduled opioid 1 month ago. He has had an excellent response according to his primary caregivers. Although not a developmentally appropriate 10-month-old, with regular opioid therapy Jake was much easier to settle, newly engaging in a social smile, and had minimal irritability with handling.

It was noted, however, that he began rubbing his cheeks into his sheets, causing significant local irritation. There is a clinical impression of increased incidence of opioid-induced urinary retention and pruritus in the pediatric population compared with the experience of caring for adults. Similarly, paradoxical reactions to such agents as benzodiazepines and antihistamines seem to appear with increased frequency in children relative to adults, but these observations are documented solely by anecdote. Jake's rubbing of the sheets with his face resolved completely with a change of opioid to hydromorphone. The other option of continuing an antihistamine was not pursued as it had negatively impacted his state of alertness and interactivity.

Consider that Jake is now 22 months old with progressive respiratory compromise. His family has elected not to pursue aggressive interventions, such as parenteral antibiotics, for treatment of his intercurrent pneumonia. Jake looks profoundly compromised, with death anticipated in hours to days. His irritability and spasticity have escalated profoundly despite appropriate titration of his analgesic regimen and antispasmodics. A discussion is held about the option of providing sedation as part of Jake's end-of-life care.

2.3.3. Pain in Children With HIV/AIDS

HIV/AIDS is known to cause pain and other symptoms from multiple causes, including the primary virus, antiretroviral treatments, and infections *(13)*. In a US-based study, 59% of the HIV-infected children reported that their pain had an impact on their life *(14)*.

2.3.4. Pain in Children With Cystic Fibrosis

There are many potential causes of pain in children with cystic fibrosis, but this is an area only recently coming to light. Among the patterns of pain, joint, head, and chest pain were noted. The causes of pain at any one site may be multifactorial, such as the relation of chest pain to a combination of osteoporosis, rib fracture, and kyphosis *(10,15)*.

3. The Assessment of a Child in Pain at the End of Life

3.1. Raising the Assessment Bar

It is widely acknowledged that pediatric pain assessment and management has lagged behind similar care for the adult population. In the last decade, the concept of addressing this aspect of care in conditions for which pain is known or presumed to be a prominent feature of the illness has been embraced. This has been notable for postoperative care, HIV/AIDS, and cancer. However, pain may still not be thought of or asked about when the child's condition is rare or poorly understood or when the emphasis is largely or exclusively focused on other aspects of care. For example, the respiratory and infectious facets of care have largely been the focus in patients living with and dying from cystic fibrosis. It is only relatively recently that the significant prevalence of pain in this patient population, including at the end of life, was described in a US chart review study *(9,10)*.

3.2. How and When to Tap Into Distress

Ill children, their parents, and the health professionals who care for them may inadvertently engage in a "don't ask, don't tell" alliance, so that the emotionally laden meaning of the child's pain, a reminder of the presence of illness and often signaling a worsening of their disease, accompanied by diagnostic tests potentially bothersome to the child can be deferred for a time. Children may not report pain because they imagine that their parents and others who care for them must know how they feel. Similarly, children and families may not report pain to the health professionals caring for the child because of a similar concept, that "the health professionals must know because they know what my child is sick with." They may also assume that if there was something to be done to address their pain, then it would have been done. Health professionals make the often-erroneous assumption that if there was a distressing symptom, surely the patient or the patient's family would inform them *(16,17)*

Although the context for this chapter is care at the end of life, continually assessing and addressing the child's pain not only is appropriate but also is a necessary component of competent care yielding great benefits throughout the child's entire illness, not just at end of life (Table 1).

3.3. Who Is the Recipient of Care?

On occasion, the health professional may be caring for a child at end of life who is deeply unresponsive, and yet the parent, family member, friend, or health professional may believe the child is "suffering." For example, the endogenous positive end-expiratory pressure (PEEP) physiological moaning pattern of breath on expiration in a dying unresponsive child may be interpreted by those

Table 1
A Checklist Template of Items to Consider for Global Pain Assessment

☑ Medication preferences
☑ Access for various routes (i.e., a central line is already *in situ* for other reasons)
☑ Preparations available (liquid, tablet, chewable, etc.)
☑ Previous experiences (positive and negative associations)
☑ Environment (i.e., medication safety in the home, history of substance abuse in child/family, neighborhood)
☑ Child's and family's information/perceptions/expectations about
  ○ Course of illness
  ○ Pain treatment, analgesics, opioids
  ○ Other
☑ Complementary and alternative therapy
☑ The child's and symptom's response
☑ Child's and family's degree of receptivity to management options
  ○ Physical measures, such as massage, acupressure, transcutaneous electrical nerve stimulation, radiotherapy (when an option)
  ○ Behavioral/cognitive techniques (i.e., guided imagery, distraction, hypnotherapy)
☑ Pharmacological management
  ○ Previous exposure, experience
  ○ Adverse effects and their management
  ○ Other effects, concerns, biases from one's life experiences (i.e., "When my Mother was dying, they gave her morphine, and she was out of it 'til her death 2 days later")
☑ Supports
  ○ Family structure
  ○ Support for the child
  ○ Formal and informal family supports, including finances, drug plan
  ○ The community of health care providers
  ○ Who is responsible for ongoing assessment and adjustment of the pain management?
  ○ Local pharmacy resources
    ○ What can and what cannot be provided in local community, hospital, or health center?
    ○ What is the usual time frame to acquire infrequently used medications (i.e., in some rural communities, from the time a prescription is written, it may take 2–3 days for a family to access the medication)?
☑ Institution-specific policies
  ○ The capacity to care for children on systemic or epidural opioids (some health centers restrict the analgesics that can be given via certain routes to certain locations of care)

(Continued)

Table 1 *(Continued)*

☑ Overall context, appropriateness for child
Pursuing the cause for the pain through diagnostic studies should be appropriate for the individual child considering the child's overall condition, what such investigations may involve in terms of travel, potential for discomfort, proximity to death, and how the results would influence the plan of care

---

present as a sign that the child is in distress. It is necessary to address this both when voiced as a concern or just silently worried about because the family is also the recipient of care in such situations.

3.4. Measuring Pain in a Child: General Principles

Measurement of pain forms one component in the broader assessment of pain. Measurement relies on a metric dimension applied to a specific aspect of the pain experience, traditionally considered in terms of intensity, frequency, or magnitude of distress. At times, assessment is made indirectly or inferred by observation of the medications used, through chart reviews noting the frequency of dosing, and doses required. The report from someone other than the child is frequently relied on for a proxy measure of pain on the child's behalf. This important task is most commonly assumed by, or falls by default to, the parent or health care professional.

Assessment includes finding out what language is used to describe pain, whether pain is talked or asked about, and in what way. Preferentially, the child is asked, or the family may act primarily in response to the child's unsolicited report. Assessment items in the history include pain location, radiation, duration, associated sensations with exposure to heat, cold, and touch, exacerbating or relieving factors, similarity to any previous episodes, impact, and impairment of usual activities of play and mobility.

It is frequently helpful to understand as much as possible about the quality of the pain. Consider the child with metastatic Ewing's sarcoma presenting with a new onset of pain in his or her right chest. The child is carefully questioned and gently examined, noting that distribution of the pain follows a radicular pattern with disturbed sensation to light touch. Such a complete picture helps the child to have confidence in the health professional and helps to validate their experience. The child appreciates that their report of pain has been both carefully listened to and believed, unfortunately sometimes not necessarily the case with the unusual pain of neuropathic origin. Such a detailed approach may also assist with diagnostic work-up, as appropriate, and help to direct the choice of pharmacological options.

3.5. Practical Pain Measurement: Self-Report Scales

The best measurement tools for a child to self-rate the severity of his or her pain have excellent practical utility and are currently the Visual Analog Scales with various facial expressions illustrated *(18,19)*. In the child 3–4 years old, a maximum of five figures satisfies the requirements that the tool be simple. In the setting of more complex patterns of pain, as in long-standing pain, semistructured interviews or a multidimensional assessment tool is more helpful, although few of the latter are available.

The developmental task required for self-report of pain with a 0–10 Likert-type scale is mastered by most children by 7 years of age. This requires an understanding of proportionality, the concept that pain is experienced by gradations within a range and anchored or limited in each direction. To then be able to apply or translate this understanding into a visual map is essential for using simple numeric or visual analog scales to self-report pain intensity *(20)*. Describing how and in what way pain is bothersome and how it may affect emotions is an abstract concept. Children who are at least 8 years old are generally able to elaborate on this *(21)*.

3.6. Pain Measurement by Methods Other Than Self-Report

Many children are unable to have their pain measured by self-report because they are nonverbal or otherwise unable to self-report by indicating nonverbally, such as by pointing. This can be because of young age, cognitive impairment, or regression with illness. The use of formal behavioral measurement scales and having a trusted caregiver report on behavioral changes observed in the infant or child are components of assessing pain in the nonverbal child. Noting changes in such physiological parameters as the elevation of pulse or blood pressure can be helpful when present. However, changes in such measures are not necessarily consistent or reliable correlates for pain, particularly in the very ill child and if pain is chronic.

One of the formal behavioral observation tools is the Gauvain-Piquard scale developed for the measurement of chronic pain in children 2–6 years old with cancer. Fifteen items have a 0–4 scale with nine items specific to pain assessment, six indicative of "psychomotor retardation," and four relating to anxiety are included in the revised version. A score greater than 12 of a possible maximum score of 60 is indicative of pain *(22)*.

3.7. Pain Measurement in Children With Neurocognitive Impairment

This patient population requires specific measures to ensure that their pain is evaluated and addressed. These children comprise a substantial number who die prematurely in childhood. Many of the life-limiting inborn errors of metabolism, such as the glycogen storage diseases, or neurodegenerative diseases have a profound impact on the child's ability to communicate both verbally or through other means.

Complicating pain assessment in these children is the fact that physical aspects of certain illnesses, such as grimacing or hypertonia, can mimic features or behaviors commonly attributed to pain. On occasion, the usual pain cues can be paradoxically manifested. For example, for the cognitively impaired child who laughs with painful procedures, such as venipunctures, laughter may be an indicator of pain.

Some of the work done in this area has provided a broader view of acute and postoperative pain. In one study, 24 children aged 3–19 years with cognitive impairment were rated by their caregivers and researchers regarding perceived intensity of the child's pain pre- and postsurgery *(23)*. One outcome of this study was that familiarity with the individual child was not necessary for observers to have congruent pain measurements *(23)*. Another study generated a checklist of "typical pain behaviors" from interviews with 33 caregivers and compared that list with another from a different cohort of 63 children with similar cognitive impairment. Seven observational items were predictive of numerical pain ratings with 85% sensitivity and 89% specificity.

It is clear that caregivers' retrospective reports may have clinical utility *(24)*. Pain cues reported by 29 caregivers of noncommunicative children 2–12 years old with life-limiting conditions were compared against a checklist of 203 items. This study yielded a common "core" set of six pain cues. These were screaming/yelling, crying, distressed facial expression, tense body, difficulty in comforting, and flinching when touched *(25)*.

Other than a singular focus on pain, there have been several tools developed for children for assessing pain, as well as other symptoms, and having these symptoms evaluated in more than one dimension. The Memorial Symptom Assessment Scale 10–18, modified from an adult version, is such a multidimensional symptom assessment tool. It was developed for children with cancer who are 10–18 years old. In a mean of 11 minutes, the majority of children were able to answer questions about how severe, frequent, and distressing they found their symptoms *(7)*. For the younger child with cancer, the scale was modified and trialed in children 7–12 years old *(11)*.

PUTTING A PRACTICAL FACE ON A CHILD IN PAIN: CASE REPORT
OF THE DEVELOPMENTAL NATURE OF PAIN ASSESSMENT

Daniel, when diagnosed with metastatic neuroblastoma at 3.5 years old, described his pain as an "owie." Following treatment with chemotherapy, radiation, surgery, and a bone marrow transplant, Daniel relapsed.

With modifications by his mother, Daniel, shown in Fig. 1 at 5.5 years old, was able to use the Faces Pain Scale to self-report pain. Daniel was unable to rate his pain with the scale when presented with all seven faces. His mother, Teresa,

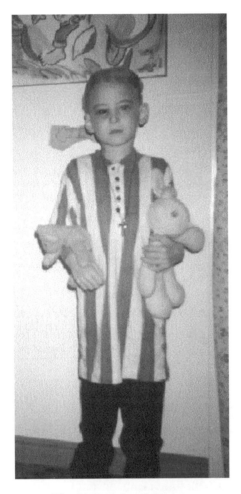

Fig. 1. Daniel at 5.5 years.

modified the scale with the tracing of his toy outline superimposed on the scale. When seeing one face at a time, Daniel could then self-rate his pain intensity on the 0–6 scale (Fig. 2) *(26)*.

The Faces Pain Scale has since been modified, tested, and validated and is now based on a denominator of 10 with representation by six faces *(19)*. This revised scale should be the one used rather than the older version shown in Daniel's story. The Web site www.painsourcebook.ca should be consulted for further details, including how to use the Faces Pain Scale–Revised in clinical practice.

4. Pain Management at the End of Life

Addressing how the child feels is central to the clinician's overall commitment to care. The fund of knowledge for providing excellence in pain management is

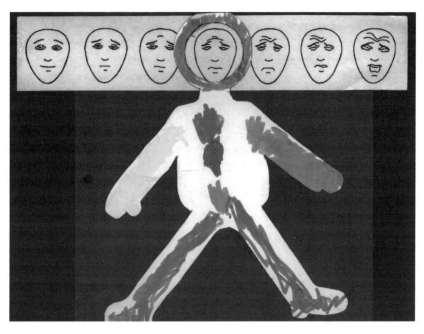

Fig. 2. The Faces Pain Scale. (Reprinted from ref. *26* with permission from the International Association for the Study of Pain.)

readily available but requires appropriate application and follow-up. This may require that the health professional reflect on and address attitudinal barriers and cultivate a willingness to seek assistance as needed. Even in the context of difficult pain management at the end of life, parents often relate how much they appreciate clinicians who remained available, showed their caring, continued to trial options for pain and symptom control, and broadly sought assistance. Parents viewed these health professionals as supportive and welcomed their efforts even when the outcome was less-than-optimal pain relief.

Pain relief with what would be considered "conventional" analgesic doses and routes is achievable for the majority of children facing pain as a consequence of advanced illness. This has been well documented in the pediatric oncology population, with the records of 199 children and young adults dying of malignancy reviewed. Only 6% of these patients required what would be considered "massive" doses of an opioid infusion, defined as 100-fold the "usual" postoperative opioid requirement *(27)*. Of that small proportion of patients, there were a few instances when "extraordinary" doses of analgesia, or the use of unusual routes, such as opioid infusions given via the subarachnoid route, or the provision of sedation was required to ensure comfort at end of life *(27)*. Similarly, regional anesthetic techniques are infrequent in treating pain at end of life for children with cancer diagnoses *(28)*. A review conducted over a 5-year period assessed the opioid doses used in children ($N = 42$) dying at a pediatric hospice. The parental morphine equivalents ranged from 0.001 to 73.9 mg/kg/hour, with a median of 0.085 mg/kg/hour *(29)*.

4.1. The Difficulty of Performing Analgesic Studies at the End of Life

The need to improve pain management in dying children is demonstrated by data that indicated that pain is often not adequately assessed and treated effectively in this population *(2)*. Improvement in pain management will be dependent not only on advances in pediatric analgesic therapeutics but also on strategies to correct the barriers to the adequate treatment of pain in these children.

There are general and specific problems peculiar to conducting analgesic studies in children. Although many of the difficulties encountered in performing analgesic trials in children can be overcome, few studies have been performed in children receiving palliative care. For example, the ethical issue of performing novel drug trials in pediatrics is somewhat mitigated by delaying such studies until the safety, efficacy, and tolerability data are available from adult studies. Similarly, obtaining the assent of a child for a drug trial, using age-appropriate explanations, mitigates the issue of only obtaining an informed consent from a proxy (usually a parent). The compromise to the problem of repeated venipuncture in children for drug assays is utilizing intravenous cannulas inserted at the time of anesthesia or blood collection from a central venous line.

Another major difficulty in performing analgesic studies in dying children pertains to the heterogeneous nature of pain in this population. Even if cancer was to be the disease model, another difficulty relates to the treatment of childhood cancer. Children tend to receive therapies directed at control of their tumors until very late in the course of their illnesses and are frequently very ill and highly symptomatic. These epidemiological and treatment variables make it less likely that a subpopulation of children receiving palliative care exists who have a stable, chronic pattern of pain amenable to evaluation in a trial. The lack of an appropriate analgesic study designed to account for small numbers of subjects is a further impediment to progress in pain management for these children.

4.2. Evidence From Analgesic Studies

Given the difficulties of performing analgesic studies in children receiving palliative care (Table 2), most pediatric analgesic studies have been performed using other pain models (e.g., postoperative pain, musculoskeletal pain, etc.). Although the pharmacokinetic and the major pharmacodynamic properties (analgesia and sedation) of most opioids have been studied in pediatrics and previously documented, little information is available about oral bioavailability, potency

Table 2
Problems Associated With Performing Analgesic Studies in Children at the End of Life

A. General issues of performing analgesic studies in children
  1. Ethical issues surrounding performing drug trials in children
  2. Consent/assent issues
  3. Practical problem of blood sampling in this population
B. Specific issues of performing analgesic studies in children with cancer at the end of life
  1. The heterogeneity of pain in children with cancer and other disease processes
  2. Lack of validated instruments to measure pain and other symptoms in children, particularly younger children, at the end of life
  3. Differences in response to and attitude toward antineoplastic therapy in children with cancer compared with the adult population
  4. Lack of a relatively stable pattern of pain
  5. The difficulties of performing drug trials in medically ill or dying children
  6. Lack of an appropriate analgesic study design that accounts for the difficulties and small patient numbers
  7. The emotional burden of caring for a dying child precludes any expectation to participate in an analgesic study

ratios, and other pharmacodynamic properties in children. In addition, there have been no controlled clinical trials of adjuvant analgesic agents in pediatrics.

4.3. Objectives of Analgesic Studies in the Context of Life-Limiting Illness

The few analgesic studies performed in the setting of life-threatening illness have been performed in the setting of pediatric cancer pain and have conformed to one of the two objectives discussed next.

4.3.1. The Evaluation of a Drug Proven Efficacious in Adult Pain Models But Now Targeted to the Pediatric Cancer Pain Population

Most of the analgesic studies of opioids performed in children with cancer *(30,31–38)* have been previously performed in adults (level 4 evidence) *(39)*. Most of the early studies had small numbers of subjects, few were controlled, and they did not use validated pain severity assessment scales. Most studies did not demonstrate differences between pediatric and adult data. Significantly, Hunt et al.'s study *(36)* demonstrated age differences in morphine pharmacokinetics compared with the adult population and recommended a starting total daily dose of morphine of 1.5–2.0 mg/kg/day to provide plasma concentrations above 12 ng/mL in children with cancer pain unrelieved by analgesics used for mild-to-moderate pain.

4.3.2. Evaluation of Novel Approaches to Opioid Delivery or Analgesic Study Design in Pediatric Population

Historically, the status of pediatric analgesic studies has improved, as have psychometric data for measures of pain severity. This has resulted in greater sophistication of pediatric analgesic studies in this patient population. For example, patient-controlled analgesia (PCA) morphine was compared with continuous infusion morphine for the relief of mucositis pain in patients aged 12–18 years. This study utilized randomized, controlled trial methodology *(40)*. Less morphine intake and fewer opioid side effects were demonstrated in the morphine PCA group (level 2 evidence) *(39)*.

Utilizing few patients, a novel pediatric analgesic study used randomized, double-blind, three-period crossover methodology *(41)*. The safety and efficacy of a clinical protocol for the administration of opioids by PCA for mucositis pain after bone marrow transplantation was demonstrated. In this small study, hydromorphone was not superior to morphine in terms of analgesia or the side effect profile. The clearances of hydromorphone and morphine in the children studied were generally greater than those previously recorded, but this finding may be related to disease or treatment variables. Apart from clearance, the morphine pharmacokinetics in the study population were similar to those previously recorded. In addition, hydromorphone may be less potent in this population of children than indicated by adult equipotency tables (level 2 evidence) *(39)*.

4.4. Clinical Care

4.4.1. Guidelines and Their Application in Practice

The majority of guidelines for pediatric pain management, where they exist, are generally focused on acute procedural or perioperative pain management. There are few to no guidelines for the management of pain in children facing the end of life related to nononcological conditions.

Disease-specific guidelines exist for palliative care for children with cancer *(1,42,43)*. It is generally not known how well such guidelines are followed, although a nationwide Swedish questionnaire surveyed all the pediatric departments about their cancer pain practices *(44)*. An astounding 100% response rate showed that most physicians (63%) followed the analgesic "ladder" approach recommended in the World Health Organization guidelines, although room for improvement was noted *(44)*. Acetaminophen or paracetamol is generally used for mild pain, representing the first step of the World Health Organization ladder. On occasion, mostly in nononcological conditions, this agent may be replaced by a nonsteroidal anti-inflammatory medication or one of the cyclo-oxygenase 2 inhibitor nonsteroidal anti-inflammatory analogs. Codeine is typically used for pain corresponding to mild-to-moderate pain. For moderate-to-severe pain, morphine is the first agent traditionally used worldwide because of access, convenience, cost, and fund of experience.

Another survey of pain practices conducted across Canada heard from 26 organizations that provide pediatric cancer care, including care in the context of palliative and end-of-life management. There were no protocols in 21% of the centers to manage the most common problems related to this aspect of care, including seizures, excessive secretions, constipation, respiratory distress, and nausea and vomiting. The difficulties in providing adequate care within the home was noted by several respondents.

A retrospective chart review was conducted evaluating end-of-life care among hospitalized children who died of HIV/AIDS in South Africa. Pain and distress in the last 48 hours was documented for 55% of the patients who died in the general wards, with a comfort care plan documented for fewer than half of the patients. Perhaps the most distressing statistic is that no analgesia was given for half of the patients with documented pain and distress *(45)*.

4.4.2. Barriers to Best Care

Much of what exists in the pediatric world literature is based on acute and perioperative studies, an empiric approach, and extrapolation from adult population studies. There is also a dearth of education preparing clinicians for the practice they face. A survey of a large organization's membership of pediatric oncologists assessed their attitudes, practices, and challenges relating to pediatric end-of-life oncological care. These individuals from across the United States, Canada, and the United Kingdom described a lack of formal courses in pediatric palliative care, great reliance on the trial-and-error method of skill acquisition, and a need for strong role models in this area. Barriers to excellence in end-of-life care and pain control care were identified as inaccessible palliative or pain services and communication difficulties between parents and oncologists *(46)*.

In the area of cognitive and behavioral interventions, sometimes globally referred to as nonpharmacological interventions for pain, there have been few consensus approaches or guidelines, but those useful for advocacy for implementation on an institutional level are available, particularly through the work of the International Society of Pediatric Oncology *(47)*. It is well recognized by many clinicians that the optimal plan of care for pain management is one that integrates both pharmacological and cognitive/behavioral approaches. Although few to no resources address the use of hypnotherapy, guided imagery, and distraction in pediatric end-of-life care, the applicable approaches are accessible through journals, books, and Web sites, with many possibilities for clinical training in these skills *(48)*.

Sadly, significant barriers persist to excellence in pediatric pain management both at the end of a child's life and through the course of the child's illness. Misperceptions and concerns relating to pain in childhood and pain relief must be proactively addressed as the child is reliant on the adult caregivers for access to measures that ensure their comfort *(17)*. Although a cross-Canada survey of pain practices in pediatric oncology centers was conducted since entering the millennium, this age of presumed increased awareness, addiction was mentioned as a barrier to optimal pain management. This mirrors the concerns clinicians encounter *(49)*.

Barriers to best management may also exist in the patient or the patient's family, as the meaning implied by reporting pain and its attendant treatment may be difficult to integrate with wishes of staying hopeful. This was poignantly reflected by one patient's comment. Ed was a thoughtful and mature 16-year-old with metastatic osteosarcoma; he generously shared his thoughts from his personal journal during what became his terminal admission. "I think the tumor is growing really fast or the swelling has gotten worse. I just can't get comfortable. Maybe I just need more drugs. I don't really want to be on more drugs. Each time I go up a drug or get a new one makes me wonder who's winning" (Frager G, personal communication, 2004).

4.5. Changing Therapeutics in the Management of Intractable Pain in Children at the End of Life: 1995–2005

Pain that cannot be alleviated using conventional treatment is intractable. Intractable pain that does not respond to therapies beyond conventional practice is refractory. The relief of refractory pain may require a therapy that reduces conscious awareness. Intractable pain in childhood is unusual and is mostly seen in the setting of cancer pain and at the end of life. Intractable childhood cancer pain is usually disease related. Disease-related pain often recurs at the time of tumor recurrence and when the cancer becomes unresponsive to treatment.

A retrospective study published in 1995 examined the opioid requirements of children with terminal malignancy *(27)*. Twelve (6%) of the patients in this study required therapies beyond conventional pediatric opioid dosing. The majority of the patients had neuropathic pain related to tumor location as the basis of their intractability. Eleven patients had spinal cord compression, solid tumor metastatic to the spinal nerve roots, nerve plexus, or large peripheral nerves. Of the patients, 50% had adequate analgesia with either regional anesthesia or high-dose opioid infusion alone. The remaining patients required the prescription of sedation to control refractory pain.

Since the publication of that report, practice has become more sophisticated, with greater understanding of the management of the pediatric pain crisis, the calculation of opioid "rescue" dosing and dose escalation, and opioid switching;

greater understanding of the management of opioid side effects to permit greater opioid dose escalation; the *N*-methyl-D-aspartate (NMDA) antagonists as new therapeutic options; and better understanding of invasive approaches to pain management in children. Given the change in therapeutics, it may be that fewer children need to be sedated to reduce conscious awareness of intractable symptoms.

4.5.1. The Pediatric Pain Crisis

The pain crisis in a dying child is an emergency and may require treatments beyond conventional means. A specific diagnosis must be made as therapies directed at the primary cause may be more effective in the longer term. The management of intractable pain requires the clinician to be at the patient's bedside to titrate incremental intravenous opioid doses every 10–15 minutes until effective analgesia has been achieved. The analgesic effect of opioids increases in a log linear function, with incremental opioid dosing required until either analgesia is achieved or somnolence occurs *(50)*.

The total amount of opioid administered to achieve this reduction in pain intensity is considered the *opioid loading dose*. A continuous infusion of opioid may need to be commenced to maintain this level of analgesia, along with "breakthrough" or "rescue" doses. In such circumstances, the initial infusion rate is often based on the opioid administered as a loading dose rather than the "usual" starting doses typically referred to in practical reference manuals *(50)*. An alternative to a continuous infusion of opioid is intermittent parenteral opioid, especially in the setting of an unpredictable pain syndrome.

4.5.2. Rescues

Breakthrough doses (or *rescues*) are additional doses of opioid incorporated into the analgesic regime to allow for additional analgesia if required by the patient. Breakthrough doses of opioid may be calculated as approx 5–10% of the total daily opioid requirement and may be administered orally every hour *(50)*. Given the frequency with which additional analgesia may be required for severe pain, it may be convenient for some children to self-administer breakthrough opioid doses using a PCA device. Data suggest that 7-year-old children of normal intelligence can use PCA effectively to provide analgesia postoperatively *(51)*.

4.5.3. Opioid Dose Escalation

If pain can be controlled by the opioid loading technique, then the subsequent opioid dose escalation may be calculated as follows:

1. If more than approximately four to six breakthrough doses of opioid are required in a 24-hour period, then the hourly average of this total daily rescue opioid should be added to the baseline opioid infusion. An alternative would be to increase the baseline infusion by 50% *(50)*.

2. Breakthrough doses are kept as a proportion of the baseline opioid infusion rate and, with dose titration, are recalculated as between 50 and 200% of the hourly basal infusion rate *(50)*.

4.5.4. Opioid Switching

The usual indication for switching to an alternative opioid is dose-limiting opioid side effects preventing opioid dose escalation. In the setting of intractability, opioid dose escalation may be limited by opioid-related side effects. An observation is that a switch from one opioid to another is often accompanied by change in the balance between analgesia and side effects *(52)*. A favorable change in opioid analgesia to side effect profile will be experienced if there is less cross tolerance at the opioid receptors mediating analgesia than at those mediating adverse effects *(53)*. In the context of refractory pain, an opioid switch may permit better analgesia with fewer opioid side effects *(54)*.

There are emerging pediatric data on the practice of opioid rotation in children with cancer *(55)*. Following a review of opioid prescription at the Children's Hospital at Westmead in Sydney, Australia, for the above indications, opioid rotation was employed in 9% of all opioid prescriptions, with a positive impact on side effect control and without a significant change in pain scores.

Following a prolonged period of regular dosing with one opioid, equivalent analgesia may be attained with a dose of a second opioid that is smaller than that calculated from an equianalgesic table. An opioid switch is usually accompanied by a reduction in the equianalgesic dose (approx 50% for short half-life opioids). In contrast to short half-life opioids, the doses of methadone required for equivalent analgesia after switching may be on the order of 10–20% of the equianalgesic dose of the previously used short half-life opioid. Protocols for methadone dose conversion and titration have been documented for adults *(56,57)*.

4.5.5. Opioid Side Effects

Children do not necessarily report opioid side effects voluntarily (e.g., constipation, pruritus, dreams, etc.) and should be asked specifically about these problems. An assessment of opioid side effects is included in an assessment of analgesic effectiveness. All opioids can potentially cause the same constellation of side effects. If opioid side effects limit opioid dose escalation, then consideration should be given to an opioid switch. Tolerance to some opioid side effects (e.g., sedation, nausea and vomiting, pruritus) often develops within the first week of starting opioids. Children do not develop tolerance to constipation, and concurrent treatment with laxatives should be provided.

There is a tendency to attribute any new adverse effects to the opioid therapy. Although warranted on occasion, it should not be assumed. Other potential causes should always be considered and ruled in or ruled out by noninvasive measures, with the temporal relationship to opioid administration and an understanding of biological and elimination half-lives all part of the equation. Adverse effects may carry greater import when occurring in children than in their adult cohort. Children do far less in the way of "bargaining" with the side effects they experience. Children live in the moment, with wishes and expectations for immediate gratification. They have little to no understanding of the cause-and-effect relationship likely contributing to their lack of patience with adverse medication-related effects despite any conferred benefit *(58)*.

Consider that a given opioid provides excellent pain relief but is making the child feel some way they dislike, such as itchy. Unlike most adults, children do not tend to understand or rationalize that sticking with it or adding another medication to reduce the pruritus will be beneficial. This tends to result in more frequent opioid rotation in children compared with adults, an observation noted in clinical experiences. To ensure ongoing trust and the child's overall comfort, any potential side effects must be anticipated and proactively managed.

Confusion can be one of the more distressing adverse effects, sometimes much more so for those close to the child than for the child as the child is sometimes unaware or distanced from awareness of his or her confusion. To lose aspects of the child's personality through medications rather than, or in addition to, illness or death is profoundly tragic. It can also frequently be prevented or ameliorated through judicious analgesic titration, opioid rotation, and the use of adjuvant therapies to widen the "therapeutic window" and minimize drug-related toxicities while ensuring pain relief.

When the confusion is attributed to opioid toxicity, whether it is idiosyncratic or dose related, the move to an alternate opioid is an appropriate one in the setting of confusion. Even if the child is unaware of his or her confusion, this kind of drastic change in the child's personality is profoundly distressing to those in attendance, the family, friends, and health professionals. However, the decision to make a change in the analgesic therapy should be based on several factors, including the expected proximity to the child's death, what the anticipated time course would be for effective pain relief with the analgesic alternative, and the attendant side effect profile. If those factors are not favorable, it may be preferable to initiate and maintain sedation until death, without agitation or other apparent distress *(59)*.

4.5.6. NMDA Receptor Antagonists

NMDA receptor antagonists depress central sensitization in animal experiments and in humans *(60–63)*. Dextromethorphan, dextrorphan, ketamine, memantine, and amantadine, among others, have been shown to have NMDA receptor antagonist activities. The clinical usefulness of some of these medications is compromised by a high ratio of adverse side effects to analgesia. There are no data of their utility in pediatrics other than for procedural pain management. Despite this, clinical usage is increasing, particularly in the setting of severe neuropathic pain and rapid opioid dose escalation and perceived tolerance.

4.5.7. Invasive Approaches to Intractable Pediatric Cancer Pain

4.5.7.1. ANESTHETIC APPROACHES

The experience of using regional anesthesia for children with intractable pain is limited. A retrospective study of children with terminal cancer (28) showed that regional anesthesia may be appropriate in a highly select subset of children. The indications for regional anesthesia in this group were mostly related to either dose-limiting side effects of opioids or relative opioid unresponsiveness in patients for whom pain was confined to one region of the body. Rapid intravenous opioid dose reduction was required in some cases (28).

4.5.7.2. NEUROSURGICAL APPROACHES

Experience with neurodestructive procedures in children is also limited, as described by the experience of cordotomy in children (64) with intractable pain. It is unclear whether these cases may now have been effectively managed by current pharmacological techniques.

4.5.7.3. OTHER PHYSICAL APPROACHES

Although prominent in clinical practice, there is little in the published literature about such modalities as radiotherapy, radiopharmaceuticals, and transcutaneous nerve stimulation, generally used concurrently with other pain management techniques. A case series reported some benefit for 29 children with symptomatic metastatic neuroblastoma sites treated with palliative radiotherapy (65). Similarly, the use of strontium-89 was reported for pain relief in children treated for metastatic disease, but the numbers were too small to be able to make any suggestions for clinical care (66).

4.5.7.4. SEDATION AS A THERAPEUTIC MODALITY FOR REFRACTORY PAIN

The use of sedation in the setting of refractory pain generally assumes that therapies beyond the conventional have been utilized, and that there is no acceptable means of providing analgesia without compromising consciousness. This trade-off between sedation and inadequate pain relief requires the consideration of the wishes of the child (as appropriate) and the child's family. The ethical issues surrounding prolonged sedation in pediatrics, including the principle of double effect, have been previously discussed (59,67,68). The continuation of high-dose opioid infusions in these circumstances is recommended to avoid situations in which a patient may have unrelieved pain but inadequate clarity to express pain perception. A variety of drugs have been used in this setting, including barbiturates, benzodiazepines, and phenothiazines *(59,67–70)*.

Acknowledgments

Grateful thanks are extended to the family of Daniel Penman, who so generously allowed their child's story and pictures to be shared. Thanks to Ed Snair, who gave permission for his journal to be read and used, and many thanks to his family for the willingness to share his journal. Jake's story is representative of the issues of children with progressive neurodegenerative illnesses but is fictitious.

References

1. World Health Organization. Cancer Pain Relief and Palliative Care in Children. Geneva: World Health Organization; 1998.
2. Wolfe J, Grier HE, Klar N, et al. Symptoms and suffering at the end of life in children with cancer. N Engl J Med 2000;342:326–333.
3. World Health Organization. The World Health Report. Geneva: World Health Organization; 1995.
4. Hongo T, Watanabe C, Okada S. Analysis of the circumstances at the end of life in children with cancer: symptoms, suffering and acceptance. Pediatr Int 2003;45: 60–64.
5. McCallum DE, Byrne P, Bruera E. How children die in hospital. J Pain Symptom Manage 2000;20:417–423.
6. Belasco J, Danz P, Drill A, Schmid W, Burkey E. Supportive care: palliative care in children, adolescents, and young adults. J Palliat Care 2000;16:39–46.
7. Collins JJ, Byrnes ME, Dunkel I, et al. The Memorial Symptom Assessment Scale (MSAS): Validation study in children aged 10–18. J Pain Symptom Manage 2000;19:363–367.
8. Drake R, Frost J, Collins JJ. The symptoms of dying children. J Pain Symptom Manage 2003;27:6–10.
9. Robinson WM, Ravilly S, Berde CB, Wohl ME. End-of-life care in cystic fibrosis. Pediatrics 1997;100:205–209.
10. Ravilly S, Robinson W, Suresh S, Wohl ME, Berde CB. Chronic pain in cystic fibrosis. Pediatrics 1996;98:741–747.
11. Collins JJ, Devine TB, Dick G, Johnson EA, Kilham HK. The measurement of symptoms in young children with cancer: the validation of the Memorial Symptom Assessment Scale in children aged 7–12. J Pain Symptom Manage 2002;23:10–16.
12. Hunt AM. A survey of signs, symptoms and symptom control in 30 terminally ill children. Dev Med Child Neurol 1990;32:347–355.
13. Oleske JM, Czarniecki L. Continuum of palliative care: lessons from caring for children infected with HIV-1. Lancet 1999;354:1287–1290.
14. Hirschfeld S, Moss H, Dragisic K, Pizzo PA. Pain in pediatric immunodeficiency virus infection: incidence and characteristics in a single-institution pilot study. Pediatrics 1996;98:449–452.

15. Massie RJ, Towns SJ, Bernard E, Chaitow J, Howman-Giles R, Van Asperen PP. The musculoskeletal complications of cystic fibrosis. J Paediatr Child Health 1998;34:467–470.

16. McGrath PJ, Frager G. Psychological barriers to optimal pain management in infants and children. Clin J Pain 1996;12:135–141.

17. Frager G, Collins JJ. Symptoms in life-limiting conditions. In: Hain R, Goldman A, Liben S, eds. Textbook of Pediatric Palliative Care. Oxford, UK: Oxford University Press; 2005.

18. Champion GD, Goodenough B, von Baeyer CL, Thomas W. Measurement of pain by self-report. In: Finley GA, McGrath PJ, eds. Measurement of Pain in Infants and Children. Seattle, WA: IASP Press; 1998:123–160.

19. Hicks CL, von Baeyer CL, Spafford P, van Korlaar I, Goodenough B. The Faces Pain Scale-Revised: toward a common metric in pediatric pain measurement. Pain 2001; 93:173–183. The website www.painsourcebook.ca should referred to for further details including how to use The Faces Pain Scale-Revised in clinical practices.

20. Collins JJ. Symptom control in life-limiting illness. In: Doyle D, Hanks GWC, Cherny NI, Calman KC, eds. Oxford Textbook of Palliative Medicine. New York: Oxford University Press; 2004:789–798.

21. Gaffney A, McGrath PJ, Dick B. Measuring pain in children: developmental and instrument issues. In: Schechter NL, Berde CB, Yaster M, eds. Pain in Infants, Children and Adolescents. Philadelphia: Lippincott, Williams, and Wilkins; 2003:128–141.

22. Gauvain-Piquard A, Rodary C, Rezvani A, Serbouti S. The development of the DEGRR: a scale to assess pain in young children. Eur J Pain 1999;3:165–176.

23. Breau LM, Finley GA, McGrath PJ, Camfield CS. Validation of the Non-communicating Children's Pain Checklist-Postoperative Version. Anesthesiology 2002;96: 523–526.

24. Breau LM, McGrath PJ, Camfield CS, Finley GA. Psychometric properties of the Non-communicating Children's Pain Checklist–Revised. Pain 2002;99:349–357.

25. Stallard P, Williams A, Velleman R, Lenton S, McGrath PJ. Brief report: behaviors identified by caregivers to detect pain in noncommunicating children. Pediatr Psychol 2002;27:209–214.

26. Bieri D, Reeve RA, Champion GD, Addicoat L, Ziegler JB. The Faces Pain Scale for the self-assessment of the severity of pain experienced by children: development, initial validation, and preliminary investigation for ratio scale properties. Pain 1990;41:139–150.

27. Collins JJ, Grier HE, Kinney HC, Berde CB. Control of severe pain in terminal pediatric malignancy. J Pediatr 1995;126:653–657.

28. Collins JJ, Grier HE, Sethna NF, Berde CB. Regional anesthesia for pain associated with terminal malignancy. Pain 1996;65:63–69.

29. Siden H, Nalewajek P. High dose opioids in pediatric palliative care. J Pain Symptom Manage 2003;25:397–399.

30. Miser AW, Moore L, Greene R. Prospective study of continuous intravenous and subcutaneous morphine infusions for therapy-related or cancer-related pain in children and young adults with cancer. Clin J Pain 1986;2:101–106.

31. Miser AW, Dothage JA, Miser JS. Continuous intravenous fentanyl for pain control in children and young adults with cancer. Clin J Pain 1987;2:101–106.

32. Miser AW, Miser JS. The use of oral methadone to control moderate and severe pain in children and young adults with malignancy. Clin J Pain 1985;1: 243–248.

33. Miser AW, Miser JS, Clark BS. Continuous intravenous infusion of morphine sulfate for control of severe pain in children with terminal malignancy. J Pediatr 1980;96:930–933.

34. Miser AW, Davis DM, Hughes CS, Mulne AF, Miser JS. Continuous subcutaneous infusion of morphine in children with cancer. Am J Dis Child 1983;137:383–385.

35. Collins JJ, Dunkel I, Gupta SK, et al. Transdermal fentanyl in children with cancer: feasibility, tolerability, and pharmacokinetic correlates. J Pediatr 1999;134:319–323.

36. Hunt AM, Joel S, Dick G, Goldman A. Population pharmacokinetics of oral morphine and its glucuronides in children receiving morphine as immediate-release liquid or sustained-release tablets. J Pediatr 1999;135:47–55.

37. Noyes M, Irving H. The use of transdermal fentanyl in pediatric oncology palliative care. Am J Hosp Palliat Care 2004;18:411–416.

38. Hunt AM, Goldman A, Devine TB, Phillips M. Transdermal fentanyl for pain relief in a paediatric palliative care population. Palliat Med 2001;15:405–412.

39. Oxford Centre for Evidence-based Medicine. Levels of evidence and grades of recommendations 2003. Available at: http://cebm.jr2.ox.ac.uk/docs/levels.htm. Accessed Jan. 2005.

40. Mackie AM, Coda BC, Hill HF. Adolescents use patient controlled analgesia effectively for relief for relief from prolonged oropharyngeal mucositis pain. Pain 1991;46:265–269.

41. Collins JJ, Geake J, Grier HE, et al. Patient-controlled analgesia for mucositis pain in children: a three-period crossover study comparing morphine and hydromorphone. J Pediatr 1996;129:722–728.

42. McGrath PA. Development of the World Health Organization Guidelines on Cancer Pain Relief and Palliative Care in Children. J Pain Symptom Manage 1996;12:87–92.

43. Berde CB, Ablin AR, Glazer J, et al. American Academy of Pediatrics: report of the subcommittee on disease-related pain in childhood cancer. Pediatrics 1990;86: 818–825.

44. Ljungman G, Kreugar A, Gordh T, Berg T, Sorensen S, Rawal N. Treatment of pain in pediatric oncology: a Swedish nationwide survey. Pain 1996;68:385–394.

45. Henley LD. End of life care in HIV-infected children who died in hospital. Dev World Bioeth 2002;2:38–54.

46. Hilden JM, Emanuel EJ, Fairclough DL, et al. Attitudes and practices among pediatric oncologists regarding end-of-life care: results of the 1998 American Society of Clinical Oncology Survey. J Clin Oncol 2001;19:205–212.

47. Masera G, Spinetta JJ, Jankovic M, et al. Guidelines for assistance to terminally ill children with cancer: a report of the SIOP Working Committee on psychosocial issues in pediatric oncology. Med Pediatr Oncol 2000;34:271–273.

48. Olness K, Gardner GG. Some guidelines for uses of hypnotherapy in pediatrics. Pediatrics 1978;62:228–233.
49. Ellis JA, McCarthy P, Hershon L, et al. Pain practices: a cross-Canada survey of pediatric oncology centers. J Ped Oncol Nurs 2003;1:26–35.
50. Cherny NI, Foley KM. Nonopioid and opioid analgesic pharmacotherapy of cancer pain. Hematol Oncol Clin North Am 1996;10:79–102.
51. Berde CB, Lehn BM, Yee JD, et al. Patient controlled analgesia in children and adolescents: a randomized, prospective comparison with intramuscular morphine for postoperative analgesia. J Pediatr 1991;118:460–466.
52. Galer BS, Coyle N, Pasternak GW, et al. Individual variability in the response to different opioids: report of five cases. Pain 1992;49:87–91.
53. Portenoy RK. Opioid tolerance and responsiveness: research findings and clinical observations. In: Gebhart GF, Hammond DI, Jensen TS, eds. Progress in Pain Research and Management. Seattle, WA: IASP Press; 1994:615–619.
54. Indelicato RA, Portenoy RK. Opiod rotation in the management of refractory cancer pain. J Clin Oncol 2003;21:87–91.
55. Drake R, Longworth J, Collins JJ. Opioid rotation in children with cancer. J Palliat Med 2004;7:419–422.
56. Inturrisi CE, Portenoy RK, Max M, Colburn WA, Foley KM. Pharmacokinetic-pharmacodynamic relationships of methadone infusions in patients with cancer pain. Clin Pharmacol Ther 1990;47:565–577.
57. Ripamonti C, Groff L, Brunelli C, et al. Switching from morphine to oral methadone in treating cancer pain: what is the equianalgesic dose ratio? J Clin Oncol 1998;16:3216–3221.
58. Frager G. Pediatric palliative care. In: Joishy SK, ed. Palliative Medicine Secrets. Philadelphia: Hanley and Belfus; 1999:157–173.
59. Kenny NP, Frager G. Refractory symptoms and terminal sedation in children: ethical issues and practical management. J Palliat Care 1996;12:40–45.
60. Eide PK, Jorum E, Stubhaug A, et al. Relief of post-herpetic neuralgia with the N-methyl-D-aspartic acid receptor antagonist ketamine: a double-blind cross-over comparison with morphine and placebo. Pain 1994;58:347–354.
61. Persson J, Axelsson G, Hallin RG, et al. Beneficial effects of ketamine in a chronic pain state with allodynia. Pain 1995;60:217–222.
62. Nelson KA, Park KM, Robinovitz E, et al. High dose dextromethorphan vs placebo in painful diabetic neuropathy and postherpetic neuralgia. Neurology 1997;48:1212–1218.
63. Eisenberg E, Pud D. Can patients with chronic neuropathic pain be cured by acute administration of the NMDA-receptor antagonist amantadine? Pain 1994;74:37–39.
64. Matson DD. Neurosurgery of Infancy and Childhood. Springfield, IL: Charles C Thomas; 1969.
65. Paulino AC. Palliative radiotherapy in children with neuroblastoma. Pediatr Hematol Oncol 2003;20:111–117.

66. Charron M, Brown M, Rowland P, Mirro J. Pain palliation with strontium-89 in children with metastatic disease. Med Pediatr Oncol 1996;26:393–396.
67. Truog RD, Berde CB, Mitchell C, Grier HE. Barbiturates in the care of the terminally ill. N Engl J Med 1992;327:1678–1682.
68. Truog RD, Burns JP, Shurin SB, Emanuel EJ. Ethical considerations in pediatric oncology. In: Pizzo PA, Poplack DG, eds. Principles and Practice of Pediatric Oncology. Philadelphia: Lippincott, Williams, and Wilikins; 2002:1411–1430.
69. Siever BA. Pain management and potentially life-shortening analgesia in the terminally ill child: the ethical implications for pediatric nurses. J Pediatr Nurs 1994;5:307–312.
70. Tobias JD. Propofol sedation for terminal care in a pediatric patient. Clin Ped 1997;36:291–293.

4

Residential Treatment Settings for Adolescent Chronic Pain Management

Rationale, Development, and Evidence

Christopher Eccleston, Hannah Connell, and Nicola Carmichael

Summary

We argue that an option for a residential treatment setting is sensible in developed health care economies. First, an analysis of the public health study of chronic pain finds that there is no good public health evidence base for any adolescent chronic pain intervention. Second, a conceptual analysis is undertaken for why removal of adolescents from their normal environments may offer a useful therapeutic option. Third, examples of current residential models, including summer camps and residential treatments, are given, and a more in-depth description is given of the Bath Pain Management Unit in the United Kingdom. Fourth, further discussion is provided on the barriers that often arise when stakeholders in children's pain services attempt to persuade each other of the importance or otherwise of intensive treatments. Finally, advice is given regarding how to develop and sustain an evidence-supported chronic pain management service for adolescents in chronic pain.

Key Words: Adolescence; chronic pain; economics; evidence; residential.

1. A Fairytale Beginning

A long, long time ago, in a land far, far away, there lived a wonderfully benevolent queen. At the start of each week, she would gather her most trusted and loyal barons and ask them what they needed to give her people health and happiness for their lifetime. Suffering, she was often heard to say, would be banished from her land, her people would know no unmanageable pain, her health care workers would know only gratitude and riches, and her name would only ever be whispered kindly on the lips of an adoring populace.

From: *Bringing Pain Relief to Children: Treatment Approaches*
Edited by: G. A. Finley, P. J. McGrath, and C. T. Chambers © Humana Press Inc., Totowa, NJ

Early one terrible morning, our queen was startled into wakefulness by an unnameable disease. A heavy cloud of dark melancholy began to gather around her. She could find no name for this feeling but knew it to be most unwelcome. Confused and in search of much-needed perspective, she climbed to the top of her tower to gaze out to the four corners of her beloved queendom. But, what met her gaze was a most terrifying sight, a sight that chilled the very blood in the chambers of her generous heart. She saw what she had feared most for all of her life, ever since she was girl playing in the gardens of organization. In a cloud of angry dust, riding at breathtaking speed, were the three "riders of health care reality." She knew as they approached, shrouded in their cloaks of obfuscation, that life would never be the same again, that choices, difficult choices, would now be her task, and disappointment the hard center of her legacy.

Who are these demons that lay waste to peaceful sleep? What could have made our queen so terrified, so lost, so suddenly disenchanted? You may know them by different names for they are mistresses of disguise. It is believed that they herald from a land called "economia principalis," and they favor the cold climates that can be found in the marshes and swamps of "jargonia" and "small print." Fear them, for they have slain much ambition and ride on the backs of horses called pride. When they come charging, they mean business. We, in our land, have come to know them by the names of resource scarcity, rational health planning, and evidence-based medicine.

2. Living With Reality

Delivering effective pain management services to children and adolescents is, unfortunately, no fairytale: there are few heroes and very few uncomplicatedly evil baddies; perhaps most importantly there are no guarantees of a happy ending. This chapter explores some of the contingencies that structure the choices made in developing effective pain services and the compromises that are often reached when health professionals (broadly defined) come to design, deliver, and maintain pain management services for children and adolescents. If there is evidence, we use it for clarification; however, if there is no evidence, just as in life, we resort to experience, judgment, and prejudice, and offer arguments that you should accept only with the necessary caution and due professional criticism.

First, we review the epidemiology of chronic pain within a public health perspective. Second, we review the reasons given for treating people away from home; the different models of care that have been attempted or are in progress are introduced. Third, we place residential treatment settings under closer scrutiny. Experience from our own setting in Bath, England, will be used as a case study to exemplify some of the issues discussed. Within this example, we develop a model of how the setting informs and structures therapy. Finally, we look critically at the production and use of evidence in the context of modern health care settings and invite debate on how evidence can best be used to bring patients into contact with effective treatment.

3. Public Health: It's for Our Own Good

In modern health care economies, service design and delivery are relatively complicated matters. Many of us have only responsibility for a small unit of care: the intervention, the patient, the ward, the drug cart, or the pain facility as a whole or maybe even the division, hospital, or region. Regardless of the size of the unit of responsibility, we are often encouraged by academics, managers with responsibilities for units larger than our own, government officers, or other stakeholders to adopt a wider understanding of the needs of the population.

For all centrally governed societies, population science is of tremendous importance. In theory, knowing the prevalence (the total number of cases present in a population in a given time) and the incidence (the number of new cases in a given time) should allow one to plan for the amount and type of resources needed to provide a viable response. In theory, if we know how many children have chronic pain within our population and how many are developing chronic pain, then we should be able to model how many will require health care provision. Similarly, if we have information on changes in incidence, then we can plan service delivery in the future. This is all relatively straightforward, then. But, how far is this realistic?

We do know how many children have chronic pain. Epidemiological studies have reported the prevalence of chronic severe pain as approx 25%, and relatively stable across a variety of developed health care economies. In a survey of 5424 Dutch children and adolescents, 54% reported experiencing pain in the last 3 months, and 25% of the overall sample reported recurrent or continuous pain for 3 months or longer *(1)*. Approximately 8% of this sample reported their pain to be intense and severe. Prevalence increased with age, and more girls than boys reported pain. Girls were more likely to report multiple pains and severe pain.

Can it really be the case that one in four of our children is suffering chronic pain? Should we perhaps surrender our current concerns and responsibilities and mobilize a campaign of action on pain? Maybe it is time to abandon science and health care provision for journalism or politics? Well, perhaps, but these data, robust across different geographic samples, should be interpreted carefully.

There is a number of issues we should take into account. First, the report of pain is a common occurrence and more frequent for girls. For example, infants at play are observed to be in pain at least three times an hour *(2)*. For a further example, a study of 1155 school-attending children (aged 6–13 years) found that 19% reported recurrent stomach pain, 23% reported weekly recurrent headache, and 18% reported back pain.

Second, many epidemiological studies, including these studies, define their terms quite precisely. For example, in the Dutch landmark study by Perquin and colleagues that has done much to draw attention to the large number of children in pain, chronic pain was not studied in the context of disability and suffering *(1)*. Although a significant minority reported chronic severe pain, all school-aged participants were attending school. For these studies, chronic pain did not equate directly with disability and suffering more broadly.

Third, just as pain severity is not always a good predictor of disability, so chronic pain is not always a good predictor of service demand, request, or use. For example, Perquin and colleagues went on to look at a subsample of chronic pain patients' requests for pain treatments over a 3-week period *(3)*. Only 31% of the sample sought the advice of a primary care physician, and only 13.9% attended a specialist pain facility. In a separate retrospective study of 195 children, half with chronic pain, they found that primary care service consultation rates were no different for the presence or absence of pain. Chronic pain alone, we argue, is insufficient to predict suffering or health care demand and utilization.

Is chronic pain a public health problem or not? The short answer is probably yes. We know that there are many children and adolescents in severe pain. However, at present we remain ignorant regarding how much pain, distress, and disability require a treatment response. Put another way, we do not know how much chronic pain reported by children and adolescents is personally or socially "acceptable." Because the relationship between chronic pain and the demand for health services is also weak, we are left somewhat in a quandary. Data on the prevalence of pain and chronic pain are insufficient for us to gauge the level of health care demand.

The focus on positive health-related behavior is also at an early stage of development. With an increased awareness of chronic pain in children and adolescents comes a flurry of theories of cause, most of which have some element of dismay at the habits of current youth. The most common concern seems to be associated with sedentary behavior. For example, walking to school *(4)* and carrying school bags *(5,6)* are frequent examples. It seems that, except in the minority of pupils who persistently carry more than 20% of their body weight, carrying backpacks alone cannot explain future disability *(7)*. Similarly, sedentary behavior alone is not associated with pain and disability. For example, in a study of adolescents, no association between objectively measured activity and back pain was found *(8)*. For a second example, a study of adolescents without pain found that the time adolescents spent watching television was also, alone, not associated with decreased physical activity *(9)*. Time spent in what they called "productive" sedentary behavior (e.g., computer homework, reading, etc.)

was associated with more physical activity. Interestingly, no one behavior alone seemed to account for either the level or the type of physical activity. Although habits of childhood may have changed, no specific change has yet been identified as a dominant risk factor for chronic pain.

We are not arguing that public health has failed completely. Indeed, there are successes. Perhaps one of the biggest successes for the reduction of risk of chronic pain has been in the related areas of disease control and accident prevention, largely enacted, respectively, through changes in the development and implementation of immunization or in transport policy and law (e.g., in some countries, traffic speed and accident prevention measures). We argue only that current epidemiology has not yet provided the data that we need to justify a public health approach to the development of chronic pain services. When we come to design and deliver services for patients with chronic pain, the population data are missing; there is no guidance on how many people have pain that is not associated with suffering and how many have disabling pain in need of treatment. Perhaps it is not yet time to abandon science for politics.

4. Leaders, Experts, and Enthusiasts

In the absence of a reliable population-based approach to chronic pain and because of the ostensibly silent problem of chronic pain in children and adolescents, the histories of new service development tend to have been idiosyncratic. We have seen a number of factors implicated in the development of new services. Perhaps the most commonly cited reason given is to "respond to local need." However, treatments have also been developed to build and maintain the reputation of expert centers, to provide the base for research, for various organizational imperatives, such as the need to use (or lose) existing resources, because a wealthy or powerful donor required it, or maybe even simply to satisfy the empire-building tendencies of individuals. In some cases, local or national guidance has had an effect, but in many cases the roots of new pain services can be traced to individual or small group action.

Chronic pain service developments are no different in this account from any other specialized services. What becomes interesting about the idiosyncratic development of different services, then, is how they fit with existing health care organizational and financial arrangements *(10)*. For example, one of the most common models of service provision is the outpatient pain clinic in a tertiary anesthesiology, rheumatology, neurology, or orthopedic care environment *(11)*. Most make use of existing organizational structures to run the pain services. Sometimes, these pain services are identified as such; other times they are part of larger acute or chronic care services.

Other service models have been developed in school settings and in primary care, and some exciting research is under way to pilot the use of technology to bring care to children with chronic pain (*see* Chapter 7). The extent to which these services can be made financially profitable, or at least resource efficient, is not to our knowledge information in the public domain. The other dominant models include summer camps for children and adolescents with chronic conditions and hospice environments for children with life-threatening and life-limiting disease, and there is a small number of inpatient and residential facilities that specialize in chronic pain management and rehabilitation.

Before turning to a closer examination of models of residential treatments, a conceptual understanding of reasons for taking patients away from their environment is needed.

5. Leaving Home Is Hard to Do

There is a popular idea that the sojourn away from one's normal environment can have therapeutic benefit. Indeed, the leisure industry is partly built on the health-restoring or health-enhancing benefits of leaving home, travel, and time spent in foreign places. On closer examination of the classic vacation, one can see that there are many factors associated with it other than the simple removal of a person from common environments.

Arguments for the therapeutic sojourn, however, are often multifactorial, not always explicit, and differ depending on the condition and the history of health care provision specific to a country or region. We have identified six main reasons for the therapeutic removal of patients from their environment: access, philosophy of care, change of context, respite and recuperation, specific environment, and therapeutic use of the environment.

5.1. Access

The first reason for treatment of patients outside the home is the same reason that we have built hospitals and treatment centers: to enable access to specialized care. The main forms of modern treatments remain pharmacological, physical, psychological, surgical, or supportive care. All of these treatments require specialized staff (who have training, supervision, and management needs), specialized procedures (e.g., drug security and management), and specialized spaces (e.g., surgical suites). The primary reason for hospitals to exist is simply as a physical solution to a problem of efficient resource allocation and effective access to quality-controlled services. Patients come to the resource.

5.2. Philosophy of Care

The second reason for treatment delivery from a particular site is that the treatment center has developed to reflect or support a particular philosophy of care. The best example of this is the hospice. Although the physical buildings are common symbols of particular hospices, it is also true that the modern hospice is typically much more than the building. For the modern hospice movement, programs of care often do not include the center, and death at home is a positive choice for many. The hospice itself, however, can be the professional home for treatment staff who share the same principles, beliefs, and model of work *(12)*.

5.3. Change of Context

The third reason for leaving the normal home environment to be treated elsewhere is to remove people from the contingencies that rigidly support ineffective, unhealthy, unsociable, or occasionally unlawful habits, and to introduce a context in which experimentation with new habits and the acquisition and reinforcement of helpful habits can occur. Just as new habits are commonly gained in new environments that may persist on return to normal environments, so being away can offer the opportunity for habit suspension, reversal, or acquisition (e.g., consider the vacation or conference). In some cases, social removal is justified in part by a focus on changing unsociable or disturbing behavior, but the removal can also serve a social order function, as a treatment of the general public in addition to the patient. This is particularly true for the isolation of contagious disease or for the removal of persons engaging in toxic, violent, or criminal behavior. Although being away from common environments does disengage people from some of the contingencies, it does not remove all, given that most are specific to each individual. Functionally equivalent influences can be recreated in a residential treatment setting that are then manipulable through treatment.

5.4. Respite and Recuperation

The fourth reason for removing people from their environment is simply to provide an opportunity for rest, respite, or recovery. The general idea is that, if the management of disease, disability, or suffering is a constant task for the patient, caregivers, or both, then the temporary reprovision of that care in a formal environment will provide opportunities for resources of time to be spent differently in the home. The typical example is respite care for families who have children with complex congenital disability caused by conditions, such as cerebral palsy.

5.5. Specific Environment

The fifth reason for treatment being situated elsewhere from the home is that there are specific factors associated with a particular environment. The best example of this, perhaps, is the spa. "Taking waters" has a long history, with arguments for the therapeutic benefits of specific water, mud, or air treatments documented from as early as pre-Roman Europe. This reason can often be extended to classes of environmental features rather than focusing on one specific geographical site. For example, there are arguments for the benefit of certain climates or for the countryside as opposed to the city.

5.6. Therapeutic Use of the Environment

The sixth and final reason is perhaps the hardest to define. Aspects of a specific environment afford opportunities for health care workers to use them for therapeutic ends. In this definition, a specific environment is not a therapeutic necessity but can be a therapeutic aid or tool. A good example could be the use of woodland or rivers for group tasks in team building during a recreational summer camp or the phrasing of a therapy task as "homework" in a school-based headache treatment. Realizing the therapeutic benefits of an environment is often dependent on the treatment philosophy, model of treatment, and the skills and experience of the therapists.

6. Models of Care

In making the above six reasons explicit, we do not mean to suggest that they are mutually exclusive or that single models of care map easily onto each of the reasons. Rather, we expect each treatment model will have a rationale based on more than one of the reasons. We suspect that the more explicit we make the rationales, the greater the clarity and therefore the easier it will be to develop new models of care. Before examining the current residential treatment programs, we first consider historical and current examples of models of residential treatment for children and adolescents. The first, following from our public health example, is the removal of people for the isolation of contagious agents and for therapeutic exposure to the elements (e.g., the sanatorium). The second is enforced social removal and subjection to treatment (e.g., the asylum). The third is the increasingly common summer camp model. Finally, we consider the residential rehabilitation facility.

6.1. The Sanatorium

Industrialization and the development of economies that depended on mass production and delivery meant that many countries in the 19th century experienced large-scale changes in population size and density. In short, many people began living in close, and poorly sanitized, proximity. When people come together, disease comes together. Tuberculosis (TB), or consumption as it was commonly known, became a major killer. Although not eradicated, it is no longer an epidemic of developed economies. However, it is of considerable historical interest for our current concern. In particular, there was a critical gap in knowledge lasting approx 60 years (from approx 1885 to 1945) between the discovery of an airborne agent *Tubercle bacillus* and the discovery of curative chemotherapeutic agents. Before the advent of curative pharmacotherapy, the major tenet of treatment for TB was the removal of the person from a community and social isolation of those with active disease. So began the brief age of the sanatorium.

The brief study of local history will, in most cases, uncover tales of the local sanatoria, and they have been the source of much romantic fiction, providing as they do an excellent setting for unusual characters and relationships (e.g., Thomas Mann's *Magic Mountain* or Haruki Murakami's *Norwegian Wood*) *(13,14)*. Much of the rationale for the sanatorium was for access to treatments, such as "fresh sea air," and clinical expertise, such as the discredited "surgical cures." However, perhaps the main rationale for social removal and isolation was as a public health measure, as a preventive treatment for the nonsymptomatic public.

6.2. The Asylum

The first known asylum for the insane was the St. Mary of Bethlehem Hospital, later named Bethlehem (or bethlem) Hospital, which bequeathed as a gift to the English language its colloquial soubriquet "bedlam." Although it has a longer history, its status as an asylum for the insane began when Henry VIII gave it royal approval in 1547.

Well into the enlightenment age, a core aspect of the treatment of the mentally ill was social removal. Although there was not a strong social contagion theory at play to justify the removal of the "distracted," there was clearly a view that removal and incarceration to protect social mores was necessary. The history of Bedlam is interesting because it offers a reflection of how mental health was understood in postenlightenment England.

Although of largely historical interest, the modern psychiatric residential facility has some resemblance to the historical example: to a large part, they exist as a method of accessing specialized resources, and critically they can provide relief and respite from punishing social settings, but they also function partly to make invisible distress and suffering and to limit social exposure to deviant and abnormal behavior.

6.3. The Hospice

The hospice is a relatively modern invention and the dedicated children's hospice an even more recent development (*see* Children's Hospice International at www.chionline.org). Pediatric hospice care is less a facility and more a philosophy for delivering care, with staff who can share the same understanding of a problem and the same skills *(15)*. There are few data on the effectiveness of the children's hospice philosophy or idea, although there seems little intrinsically wrong with the concept of multidisciplinary expert care for the management of end of life and death. However, there are now good data on the assessment of the needs of children, adolescents, and their families in maximizing the quality of remaining life and managing death, grief, and loss. In particular, data from families at Canuck Place in British Columbia, Canada, found substantial need for a dedicated facility for patients and after provision found that families reported significant support for such a dedicated facility *(16,17)*.

At present, we have data on good examples of hospice programs but lack larger-scale survey or review data. An interesting systematic review of adult palliative care, for example, reported on the overall need and provision of palliative care facilities and found that, in particular, the management of pain remained a significant un-met need *(18)*. Chapter 3 in this volume refers in more detail to the provision of pain management at the end of life.

6.4. The Summer Camp

Traditionally, camps for children with chronic illness have been seen as a form of recreation for patients and respite for caregivers. There are, of course, health benefits to recreation. Adolescents with low social involvement and activity engagement are thought to be at risk for greater mental health problems. For example, one study investigated the involvement of adolescents in afterschool organized activity and found that those with low involvement also experienced greater depressed mood *(19)*. This was especially true for those with detached relations with parents. Interestingly, for this study, the engagement with the activity leader was a strong determinant for positive outcomes. More involvement in structured outdoor activities is of general benefit and can help overcome barriers to exercise and activity engagement, especially for girls *(20)*. Many children with chronic illness have reduced opportunities for social engagement, leisure, and play. The camp was a simple idea to provide the opportunity for access to leisure with expertise. Often, camps also enabled opportunities for socialization with children experiencing similar problems and opportunities for other family members (e.g., siblings) to be exposed to shared experience. In addition, it is sometimes argued that the camp provides "time-out" from stressful habits and home routines.

There has been a move to view the camp as a potential method for targeting psychosocial and educational interventions aimed specifically at adjustment. Moving beyond shared experience and recreation, some camps have more programmatic and structured content aimed at facilitating or promoting adjustment to chronic illness. There are now camping programs for mixed groups of children with different chronic illnesses and camps that are for specific client groups. The number of specialized camps has increased in the last 20 years, and there are now many camps, particularly in the United States, for children with, for example, asthma, renal disease, burns, cancer, diabetes, obesity, or arthritis.

Plante and colleagues, in a review of group interventions for pediatric chronic conditions, specifically reviewed the literature on summer camps *(21)*. They identified 23 reports of camps that ranged from day or residential camps. In some, the content offered was purely recreational activity; in others, there were clear psychoeducational components. In this overall review, they included all of the studies they could find regardless of quality. Many of the studies were case reports and uncontrolled evaluations, although some investigators had made attempts to control for variables other than the camp-delivered experience. Plante et al.'s overall conclusion was that "pre-post evaluations have indicated that campers gain disease-related knowledge and may have improvements in self-esteem, anxiety, attitudes toward the illness, and management of asthma, diabetes, and obesity" (p. 442), but they cautioned against strong statements regarding the efficacy of these interventions because of the variable and uncontrolled nature of the studies.

In attempting to focus on outcomes, in 2004 Kiernan et al. updated the review of the efficacy of camps, finding much the same result: there may be therapeutic benefits over and above recreation and respite, but they are certainly not global and are inconsistent across camps *(22)*. They therefore undertook an analysis of one large European camp program. The Barretstown Gang camp was founded in Ireland and was based on the Hole in the Wall Gang camps in the United States. This 10-day summer camp was designed for children (or siblings) with life-threatening illness and takes children from all over Europe. They were able to include 240 campers who completed the precamp assessment, and recovered data from 151 immediately postcamp and 119 at 3-month follow-up. The content of the camp was largely recreational and educational. Their findings are worth closer evaluation. They found that younger children gained more benefit from the program in physical symptoms and increases in positive affect. They also found that adolescents reported increases in judgments about quality of life at 3 months postcamp. However, and it is an important qualifier, there were examples of adverse effects immediately postprogram that were thought to be associated with friendship relationships, particularly for some adolescents, an increase in dissatisfaction with physical appearance, and immediate postcamp loss in quality of life, thought to be associated with the sudden drop in social support.

As with any complex intervention that argues for therapeutic status, the responsibility is on the providers to identify and control the therapeutic agent. The question arises regarding whether it is the general landscape of therapy that is crucially important, some aspect of the therapy (e.g., group treatment, the location, the components, the facilitator, etc.), or the content of the treatment specifically. This research has not been undertaken. To date, we do not know if there is anything therapeutic about the specific aspects of being in a camp, such as the country environment, the use of the summer camp model (e.g., in the language), the focus on leisure, recreation, and fun, the focus on friendship and support, the expert facilitation, or any specific combination of these.

6.5. The Residential Treatment Program for Adolescents

In well-established health care systems, there is a general lack of understanding of the needs of adolescents in comparison with those of adults or children. Often, these needs are discussed in terms of "transition of care" between traditional models of adult or child therapy provision, although other models are available (23,24). In many countries (the United Kingdom is a good example), the development of adolescent medicine as a specialty or subspecialty has been slow. Similarly, although there is a cogent argument for the benefit of dedicated assessment and treatment programs or centers for adolescents, their development has been equally slow or is in decline.

Although, when asked, adolescents report specific health concerns and that they would like different points of contact for health care advice than commonly exist, there are few examples in primary or secondary care of programs of adolescent health delivery (25). In tertiary care, there is also a lack of dedicated facility for adolescents with chronic or recurrent medical problems. For example, a UK survey identified that only 9 of 225 responding hospitals supported specific general adolescent medical facilities, and only a quarter had dedicated adolescent facilities or staff of any kind (26).

Given that centers of adolescent medicine are relatively rare, rarer still is the specialized center or treatment program for adolescents with chronic pain. There are good examples internationally of pediatric pain leaders winning and maintaining access to, or control over, general medical beds or delivering outpatient multidisciplinary pain management programs, but unusual is the dedicated residential program of treatments.

A pioneer of this type of treatment program is David Sherry, a pediatric rheumatologist. Dr. Sherry and colleagues identified that the typical response of modern health care systems to an adolescent chronic pain problem was not achieving the desired outcome and in some cases may have contributed to suffering. He identified that a large number of children presented to outpatient pain or rheumatology clinics with complex regional pain syndrome type (CRPS)-1 (also known as reflex sympathetic dystrophy or algodystrophy). Adolescents typically present with a limb (usually foot or hand) that is the object of intense pain, hyperalgesia, and trophic adaptation. Patients, on assessment, are often fearful and depressed. Typically, they refuse to bear weight on the affected limb and have become, or are quickly becoming, disabled.

The optimal treatment for recovery from CRPS-1, and prevention of further disability, is early exposure to high-dose self-initiated and self-maintained physiotherapy. Typically, however, health care organizations are not structured in a way that easily enables this model of treatment. To increase access to high-dose appropriate physical therapy, Dr. Sherry developed a residential model of treatment in which a multidisciplinary team of physiotherapists, occupational therapists, social workers, nurses, and physicians could work on the same consistent and comprehensive treatment philosophy and model. To access this specific model of treatment in the appropriate doses, the patients are required to be residents in the hospital, hotel, or a private accommodation. The proximity to the therapy team allows reliable access to treatment.

Adolescents and their parents are referred for assessment at the Children's Hospital of Philadelphia. If accepted onto a treatment program, they work individually with a specialist team and are exposed to physical and occupational therapy for an average of 6 hours a day for an average of 14 days over 3 weeks. The therapy is aimed at reactivation, movement of the affected limb, exposure to pain on movement, desensitization, and reinforcement of exercise and activity engagement. Given the high dose of exposure to pain-inducing treatment, maintaining engagement is a major therapeutic challenge. Creativity in the choice of exercises and methods of maintaining compliance are, in this therapy, crucial to treatment success. The therapists have developed a range of tasks and techniques to maximize engagement. Therapist skill and adherence to a "counterintuitive" but clinically appropriate model is paramount to the success of the treatment.

Outcome data on 103 patients showed that 92% of children were symptom-free immediately postprogram. Only half of the sample was available for follow-up. Of these, 88% remained symptom-free at 2 years *(27)*. Although there are significant problems of a relatively high degree of selectivity and dropout in these evaluation studies, with a lack of knowledge regarding how many adolescents with chronic pain were not able to enter or maintain treatment, the overall picture is promising. In one of the most disabling and clinically confusing chronic pain conditions, CRPS-1, it is possible to effect large and meaningful changes in symptom reduction and function. Multidisciplinary rehabilitation is a promising therapy for adolescent chronic musculoskeletal pain, and some have argued that maybe the only viable response to a multidimensional and chronic problem of widespread disability and pain is a comprehensive multidisciplinary one *(28–30)*.

7. The Bath Pain Management Unit

The Bath Pain Management Unit is, organizationally, one-third of the Royal National Hospital for Rheumatic Diseases, National Health Service Trust. The small national hospital provides specialized services in chronic pain, rheumatic diseases, and neurorehabilitation. It is housed on the site of the original Roman

Spa and was built as a specialized hospital in 1742; originally called the Mineral Water Hospital, it was later renamed the Royal National Hospital for Rheumatic Diseases *(31)*.

In 1993, two senior rheumatologists identified that they needed to develop rehabilitation for adults with chronic pain and invited the first author to consult on its development. The Pain Management Unit (PMU) was developed to deliver specialist assessment of adults with chronic pain and a 3-week residential treatment program for adults with chronic pain *(32)*. The PMU soon became self-governing and was organized, and remains organized, around a central principal encapsulated in its vision statement: "to enable people to reduce the impact of pain on their lives, and to influence society's attitude to pain."

In 1998, a number of events collided with a serendipitous result. First, the PMU began to receive referrals for patients who were under the age of 18 years. Second, analysis of the adult assessment data revealed that 10% of the adults reported that their chronic pain had started in their childhood or adolescence, but they had not had access to treatment until adulthood. Finally, a visiting pediatric professor provoked us to change the much-loved vision statement or take up the real challenge: to treat a wider age range of people. A clinical development plan and a business plan were developed to support a new service. Adolescents with chronic pain are referred from all over the United Kingdom for assessment in a joint pediatric rheumatology and psychology outpatient clinic. If appropriate for treatment, they are referred, subject to funding approval from their local health authority, to the residential program.

8. Bath Pain Management Program

8.1. Treatment Environment

The current physical environment is spread across three adjacent sites. First, patients and parents are resident in a top-floor apartment complex adjacent, but unconnected, to the hospital. This is long-leased by the PMU for this purpose and is a nonclinical environment; half the complex is rented on a commercial basis to nonpatient customers. Second, the pain management unit, where staff has offices, is located on the third floor of the main hospital building. Currently, two therapy spaces and office accommodation are available. Third, much of the physical therapy takes place in a local public gym. All of these three therapy spaces are located in the center of Bath, a busy tourist city in southwest England. There is a further office complex on the university site where dedicated research staff are housed, but patients do not use this site.

8.2. Treatment Structure

The pain management program is delivered to groups of six young people aged between 11 and 18 years. (The full age span is often present in each group.)

An adult accompanies each young person. The adult has two tasks. The first task is to act as the guardian for the adolescent. This also means that the service provider, the hospital, does not have to be staffed with pediatric nurses to act as a guardian for the children, giving the environment more in common with home and school than a hospital ward and substantially reducing costs. The second is to enable the primary caregiver of the adolescent to be exposed to treatment. This has become more explicit as an aim over the history of the treatment. The accompanying adult, usually the mother (although we have had good results with grandparents and older siblings), is present during most of the therapy sessions and is expected to participate in group discussion, exercise, and activity sessions.

Because patients are treated in groups of six, this means that therapy sessions are often taken in groups of 12 people (six adolescent–adult dyads) or 2 parallel sessions of 6 adolescents and 6 adults. During the course of the program, how people relate to one another is closely observed within each dyad and group and between group and team. This provides valuable clinical material.

The reactions of the group members to program demands are another source of therapeutic material. Similarly, the frustration of adolescents or parents frustrated with their situation, and the expression of this, is important to identify. These situations can be supported and more useful ways of interacting and dealing with the problem found. The intensive residential environment allows for their frequent occurrence, for the consequences of the behavior to occur also in the environment and to be addressed immediately or without substantial delay. This leads to the therapy occurring at a faster pace, providing quick successes to the group, which reinforces change.

A further strength of group work is that, over the course of the process of therapy, exposure to others with similar and dissimilar experiences can have therapeutic value within a managed environment. For only one example, in early stages of therapy, patients and parents who typically have been isolated with a chronic problem are able to share experience and hence have their chronic (mis)understanding of a problem challenged.

Treating the young people in groups provides useful developmental information. In the group setting, opportunities to observe the adolescents and their parents in normal social situations rather than in the shorter intense therapeutic relationship occur. This allows the team to identify other developmental issues that may make change more difficult for certain children. An example is the observation of poor social skills or awkward peer interactions. If this is occurring in the therapeutic group, then it will also be happening at school and will need to be addressed if the young person is to return successfully to education. Specific learning difficulties that may interfere with the management of pain can also be observed during the therapeutic tasks, for example, poor sequencing and problem solving or writing difficulties that may suggest dyslexia or dyspraxia, to name but a few.

8.3. Interdisciplinary Team

The therapy team consists of a senior nurse, physiotherapist, occupational therapist, consultant pediatric rheumatologist, and consultant clinical psychologist. Research officers and students also work in support of programs. Assessment and access to the program are managed in a joint rheumatology/psychology clinic. In the program, the team operates in a thematic interdisciplinary model in which skill sharing and task crossover are encouraged (within professional limits). The process is managed by the clinical psychologist. A larger backup team exists in the unit; this team consists of other clinical staff working on adult programs, office staff working on maintaining communications or securing financial support for treatment, and research staff developing research on the measurement of chronic pain and on effective treatments for chronic pain.

8.4. Therapy Philosophy and Content

The core philosophy of the program is to promote developmentally appropriate behavior and normal health behavior despite chronic pain. For narrative purposes, the program is described as having three main themes.

First, patients are exposed to education on disease, pain, and pain-related behavior in self and others. Time is taken to assess and make sense of belief systems as they relate to diagnosis, prognosis, medication beliefs, and attitudes. In particular, patients and adults are encouraged to be explicit about their beliefs and images about pain and what is happening in their bodies. Sharing different understandings between group members is also encouraged. Discussion of how different understandings are developed and become rigidly adhered to is introduced within a therapeutic frame.

Second, return to developmentally appropriate activity is encouraged by increasing fitness and mobility, managing activity, rediscovering what was and can be valued in life, and developing methods of overcoming barriers to achieving valued activities. It is therefore important that the goals the young person has are ones that serve the person to do what he or she wants and is not imposed by others (parents, peers, or therapy staff). For example, walking 25 m may be a dull and pointless task to an adolescent, but walking to a café with friends is an age-appropriate social and physical task that increases the possibility that the goal of walking 25 m is accomplished. Physical conditioning is also a core part of the program. However, physical exercise is undertaken in a number of settings to overcome the development of site-specific exercise behavior. Patients exercise in a room with no equipment, in their bedrooms, in a pool, and in a public gym where they share the space with other gym users. By not using hospital facilities, the young people are exposed to the benefits and difficulties of the space that they will be using at home and can be supported in overcoming these difficulties *(33)*.

Third, there is a focus on the management of mood and emotion, the identification and promotion of value-based behavior, and a focus on the rigid investment in specific beliefs about the causes and consequences of pain. Most of the emotional management methods arise from a tradition within cognitive behavior therapy *(34)*. More recently, however, the clinical work has been evolving to embrace more of the work developed in acceptance and commitment therapy *(35,36)* and contextual cognitive behavior therapy *(37)*. There is a number of different interventions interweaved across the therapy in this more psychological component. For illustrative reasons, we focus on three.

The first therapeutic intervention arises from acceptance and commitment therapy and is known as *creative hopelessness*, in which young people recognize the solutions to their problems that have worked and the attempted solutions that have not worked *(35)*. This intervention must be honest and open, and the clinicians need to be able to expect and understand the expression of strong emotion as young people realize the futility of some of their past strategies, such as resting until the pain goes away.

Next, the adolescent connects with the type of lifestyle he or she wishes to lead and currently is not leading because of the impact of pain. By exposing adolescents to the values they hold about life, reasons for working hard and making changes are found. Return to school, for example, is not just pursued as necessary for statutory or regulatory reasons. The value of formal education for achieving personal values, whether learning in its own right or as a means to be able to contribute to society or provide financial support for the adolescent's own hoped-for future, is allowed to emerge as a reason for reengagement. Return to school is also desirable because of the opportunity for exposure to normal age-appropriate adolescent behavior.

The second form of intervention is aimed at coming in contact with negative aversive thoughts and emotions. Group members are encouraged to recognize thoughts as just that—thoughts—and not as unchallengeable expressions of reality. A defusion of the thought from the strong belief that the thought must be real and a reason to direct behavior is the ultimate goal. The adolescents are encouraged to become aware of their feelings and bodily reactions and to generate alternative strategies to their habitual ones.

A useful tool here is, for example, a "hot head, cool head" thought examination procedure. Hot-head thoughts are immediate reactions to situations or catastrophic developments in the mind, such as "I can't exercise; it will injure me, and then I will have to use a wheelchair." These keep the young person fixed in a status quo. Cool-head thoughts are the more useful thoughts that enable a young person to move forward and make "smart choices" or good decisions. This whole intervention is done with little talking and as much doing as possible. This gives the group members real experiences of what the dyads need to be able to transfer to home. This task is not performed within a context of mental hygiene or a focus on what are good and bad thoughts; rather, the focus is on the identification of thoughts as thoughts that can bring unwanted and aversive consequences *(34)*.

The third form of intervention is based on a mindfulness extension of traditional pain management relaxation. Again, for reasons that are beyond the limits of this chapter, relaxation has been largely replaced by mindfulness in this approach to chronic pain *(38)*. By developing the skill of noticing but not reacting to the thoughts, physical sensations and emotions that are experienced moment by moment, cognitive vulnerability to stress, and emotional distress are reduced *(39)*. The evidence base for relaxation in recurrent and acute childhood pain (particularly headache) is excellent for reducing the severity and frequency of episodes of pain *(40)*. Mindfulness often has the side effect of relaxation, but it is more useful in chronic pain as a method for enabling people to experience unpleasant body sensations, thoughts, or emotions but not allow these experiences to dominate and overshadow the good parts of their life, a core aim of the therapeutic intervention.

8.5. Therapy Process

The therapy operates by a standard process of change that is used as a model by the team to monitor therapy progress. For week 1, the process involves adaptation to the new environment, learning of new understandings of chronic pain, experimentation with different ways of thinking about thinking, behaving in pain, focusing on the relationships with significant others, and exposure to painful exercise within a graded activity and reinforcement program.

For week 2, parents and adolescents are separated for much of the therapy and follow separate tracks. Week 2 is when difficult ideas are reinvestigated, easily acquired behaviors become fragile, and sustained behavior change requires practice. Typically, patients are tired, having increased radically their uptime; easy changes have been achieved; and habit reversal and formation become challenging.

Week 3 focuses on consolidating changes that have been made and making plans for the short and long term. Commitment to continue with pain management at home is established and developed. Adults and young people reform a close functional relationship, and a model of shared family problem solving is developed. Familiarity with the process of change of dyads and groups means that atypical patterns can be challenged to ensure maximum benefit from the intervention.

8.6. Evidence of Effectiveness

The results of the first cohort of patients entering and completing this treatment have been published *(41)*. We reported on the first 57 dyads (adolescent patient and accompanying parent) entering the treatment program and the 43 who returned to follow-up at 3 months posttreatment. Data were collected from both patients and adolescents immediately pretreatment, posttreatment, and 3 months following treatment. Data were also taken at 12 months following treatment but are not yet available.

Of the 57 patients entering treatment, 41 were female. The most common diagnosis was of CRPS-1, and the average chronicity was 4 years. Most patients reported their pain to be persistent, and the average pain severity was relatively severe at 6.69 (range 1–10). Most of the adolescents were not in formal education because of pain, and the average amount of time away from full-time education was 17 months (with a median of 12 months). The adolescents were referred from a wide geographical area in the United Kingdom, most commonly by pediatric musculoskeletal specialists at children's hospitals in the United Kingdom or by community pediatricians.

Adolescents completed a battery of physical performance measures, including the number of sit-to-stand movements they could make in a minute and the speed of walking over a 10-m distance. They also completed self-report questionnaires on a range of psychosocial domains, including pain depression, anxiety, coping efforts, disability, somatic awareness, and school attendance. Parents also completed self-report measures about their own anxiety and depression and the parenting stress index that assesses the extent and type of stress they experience in the parenting role. The parents also completed measures of their child's pain, depression, and disability.

Immediately postprogram, the data showed that the children reported no difference in pain, anxiety, depression, coping, or somatic awareness, but they could sit to stand more times within 1 minute, and they could walk more quickly. Analysis of the 3-month data, however, showed that the children made significant gains on returning to the home environment. Importantly, they reported less anxiety and anxious coping, less awareness of their bodily sensation, and less disability. The gains they had made on physical performance were maintained. Therefore, the adolescents showed an interesting pattern, somewhat similar to the camp study reported in Subheading 6.4., in which the greatest benefits are seen at some time following the programs *(22)*.

Analysis of the parental data showed a different pattern. First, parents reported that they did see improvement in their child's disability immediately postprogram. Second, they reported immediately postprogram that they themselves were less depressed, less anxious, less aware of their own physical symptoms, and much less stressed about how to parent their child. All of these significant parental gains were maintained at 3 months following treatment. Although we have been able to establish a link between adolescent depression and parenting stress in this sample, the data set is still too small to answer the interesting question of the relationship between parental therapeutic gain during the program and its putative effects on adolescent change following the program *(42)*. However, given the focus in this therapy on parent involvement and the recognition of the effects of parental distress and parental coping on child coping, we expect a relationship to emerge between parent change and child change.

The two most intriguing findings from this research refer to child behavior. First, across all stages of measurement, the adolescents reported no significant reduction in pain. However, there were significant changes in function and disability at posttreatment and greater improvements at 3 months following treatment. The stability of pain as a complaint is not unusual, is a common finding in the adult literature, and should be understood within the context of this treatment, which does not have pain relief as a goal *(43)*. The breakdown in the relationship between pain and function is at the heart of this therapy. Patients and parents are aiming to live toward their valued goals in spite of pain. Pain becomes an invalid reason to reduce function.

Second, in addition to self- and parent report data, we also routinely collect school attendance data. Returning adolescents to normal social environments is an important goal of therapy. At the beginning of the therapy only 14 adolescents were in full-time education; following treatment, 29 were in full-time education. Because some of the adolescents had already left school or were already in full-time education, improvement was only possible for 42 patients. After controlling for this ceiling effect, the data showed that 27 increased their exposure to formal schooling, 12 remained the same, and 3 reduced their exposure. Analyzing the data as a sample in terms of amount of time spent, there was a significant increase in the number of half days of school attended (1–10), from a mean of 3.28 before treatment to a mean of 5.69 at 3 months.

In this small sample of complexly disabled patients who have reported pain and disability for an average of 4 years and referred nationally to a specialized pain program, it is possible to achieve significant change in function and disability-related behaviors, including return to normal environments, despite pain. Emerging as potentially crucially important in the maintenance and extension of improvements in the long term are improvements in parenting stress and parental mental health during treatment. More study of the relationship between changes in parental variables and their putative effects on change in adolescent variables is necessary. If there were to be an epidemiological survey of pain undertaken in school settings now, these patients may well report their pain as high. However, we would argue, as might the patients, that this high pain does not equate with suffering or disability.

9. The Darkening Skies

We have reviewed the evidence for the effectiveness of at least two instantiations of multidisciplinary chronic pain rehabilitation delivered in a residential setting and reported it to be promising. Adolescents with long-standing, resilient, severe pain and complex disability can make statistically significant and clinically meaningful changes, returning in many cases to normal function.

However, and it is a big however, there is no evidence for the comparative advantage of any one model of delivery over any other model of delivery. There have been no randomized controlled trials (RCTs) of residential vs nonresidential, of summer camp vs hospital treatment, of hospice care vs nonhospice care at end of life, or of health restorative benefits of the beaches of Nova Scotia vs the beaches of British Columbia.

Lack of evidence is not, of course, the same as evidence against effectiveness. Does the lack of these comparative studies constitute a flaw in the evidence base? Is this absence a cause for major concern? From a certain point of view, the answers must be yes. However, there are other points of view, other stakeholders who need to bring evidence to bear. Indeed, there is what can best be described as a nervous system of forces in multiple simultaneous opposition, rarely in balance, with rarely the same stakeholder's views winning. Fonagy and colleagues reminded us of the often-opposing perspectives of four of the stakeholders in the production and use of evidence *(44)*.

9.1. Researchers

The research process is applied to answer questions that not only arise from clinical environments (e.g., is a particular treatment effective?) but also are often driven by a combination of intellectual interest, philosophical investments, and funding priorities. How questions are phrased and answered is shaped by a variety of features, including established methodological practice, habit, and statistical procedures. The main aim of the research process is to isolate and define key variables that lead to change. Part of the process is to identify and control the effects of the multiple changing variables, either in research design or in statistical procedures. Often, what is the richness and variability of patients' lives becomes managed as "statistical error." Outcomes are commonly reported as average changes of samples of populations or as probabilities for therapeutic or adverse effects.

9.2. Clinicians

The clinical process of working with children with long-term conditions is complex. Clinicians are often aware of multiple interacting variables that can affect change and use these variables as important parts of formulation and treatment. Treatments are normally driven by available resources, staff, their skills, and space, and financial support. Diagnosis is often unhelpful to the clinician in the therapy process with chronic pain because it offers little guidance, and individualization of the therapy is often necessary. Outcomes are commonly individualistic, based on agreed outcomes that are relevant and important for the patient and that are driven by the therapy rationale. Outcomes are rarely calculated in percentages and are often normatively related. Importantly, acceptable outcomes to patients are often the subject of therapy and can change in the process (e.g., from pain relief to greater functioning with pain).

If measurable outcomes are used, then they relate to a range of functional abilities that may be restricted by pain, not purely to the level of pain, although this is the headline purpose of referral for assessment and treatment and the common parlance of funding discussions.

9.3. Patients

Children and their parents are concerned typically with their own experiences, with the realistic and well-founded fear of future aversive experience, and with gaining access to treatment. Potential outcomes are not perceived in terms of group average data or probabilities of good outcomes, and they are not conceived in terms of cost-efficiency of the available resources. Instead, they are highly individualized, and in chronic pain are often focused on single goals, such as relief from pain. Depending on the source of funding, patients do not always understand the costs of treatment or the opportunity costs of the investments in their treatment (i.e., that in funding this treatment other treatments for other people may not be funded).

9.4. Funders

The funding process is driven by the need to match resource to need equitably within a context of resource scarcity and the relative value of treatment outcome. This complicated situation is often discussed under the rubric of cost-effectiveness. When a decision is made and held regarding the value and utility of a treatment, the aim is for its provision to be as cost-effective as possible so that the lowest possible unit of resource can be invested to produce the highest possible outcome. Research can often give an idea about the potential value of a treatment, and clinicians can speak eloquently to the need to account for multiplicity and to individualize treatments, but these do not necessarily inform judgments about appropriate investment and acceptable local cost-efficiency or are not always presented in a language that is understood by funders.

In the United Kingdom, evidence-based health commissioning is slowly evolving through the implementation of centralized initiatives (e.g., National Service frameworks and clinical effectiveness guidelines). The number of such frameworks and guidelines remains small, and for the most, part health care rationing is not undertaken rationally. In particular, there is rarely any attempt to assess the values, and willingness to pay, of a population for any given condition or for a choice of treatment across conditions.

When funders are asked to consider commissioning residential interventions for pain, it should not be assumed that the clinical consideration of an individual's level of complex disability is transparent to them. In the absence of any national agreement to address complex disability and pain, when deciding whether to fund such interventions, funders will rely on their broad knowledge of population norms for pain and their experience of the dominant understanding of pain as a disease-related and a simple treatment problem. Therefore, in this case, the common comparison is with uncomplicated pain that can be treated on an outpatient or community basis (the bulk of our 25% of children reporting pain). In the context of a larger commissioning framework, it will always be difficult to argue for the clinical effectiveness or cost-effectiveness of residential treatment because there is rarely a shared language of need, of the potential benefits of treatments to patients and to society at large, or for that matter, the costs of failing to treat.

10. Using Evidence to Bring Patients Into Contact With Potentially Effective Treatment

Not all treatments need RCTs to form the evidence base. Some of the most commonly used and effective treatments lack trial data. In addition, some treatments have no proven effectiveness, but their withdrawal would result in no treatment, creating a socially intolerable vacuum in service provision and the destruction of an environment in which potentially effective treatments could be developed. Consider, for example, the proposal that hospice services should be withdrawn for lack of RCT evidence.

When evidence is called for, it is usually because one of the above stakeholders has a concern: the clinician has developed a new or variant approach, the researcher is interested in establishing differences from other approaches, the funder is responding to requests to spend limited resources differently, or the patient has multiple unmet needs. When evidence is called for, it will be important to remember that, given the opposing positions of stakeholders, evidence is likely to become contentious and will nearly always be challenged by one of the stakeholders. In short, no one piece of evidence or review of evidence, however systematic, will win all arguments.

To use evidence to its best effect and to bring patients into contact with treatment, it is necessary to develop a shared understanding by all stakeholders. We have identified that clinicians and patients adopt a highly individualized view and may have complex objectives for rehabilitation. Funders, however, generally adopt a population and normative approach. What often quickly becomes a problem is that there is no clearly defined and agreed definition of a subpopulation of pain management patients requiring more intensive intervention. In this context, there is rarely any agreement between stakeholders on the basis for reaching a decision. Therefore, tensions and conflicts may arise, often because the lack of understanding of different stakeholder positions and philosophies turns into questioning of personal skills or motives. In the United Kingdom, a recognition of the general failure of commissioning has led to the reintroduction of commissioning led by the general practitioner in an attempt to put a clinical voice at the center of these decisions.

Important in bringing patients closer to treatment will be the development of a critical understanding of evidence-based medicine, its uses and abuses, its benefits, and its shortcomings. Slavish allegiance to any one perspective runs the risk of moving patients further away from treatment by alienating key stakeholders with the influence to bring about effective treatment. When centers or leaders have been most successful is when they have developed an evidence-supported position for patient need, economic value, clinical effectiveness, and patient satisfaction and have engaged all stakeholders.

11. And They All Lived Happily Ever After

All good fairytales end "happily ever after," don't they? Well, no, not always. Angela Carter reminded us that fairytales, even the ones with happy endings, always betray a hidden darker version of reality *(45)*. Subtexts are nearly always also found that speak of secrets, shame, and lies; of villains and weaklings dispatched without justice; of hegemonic patriarchal morality banishing precocious attempts at usurpery; and perhaps most pertinent to the current arguments, of grief and loss. Models of delivery of chronic pain management will come and go. In the absence of a strong public health argument for coordinated widespread treatment programs for adolescents with chronic pain, treatments will develop in isolated pockets, driven often by individuals, in temporarily supportive environments. What is missing, however, is any widespread change in the overall system to embrace these treatments as a standard or as a requirement. We are too often debating in response to the question: should we support the provision of this treatment? We argue that whenever this question is proposed, before answering one should pause to consider the following alternative questions. How is it possible that this question could ever be asked? From which understanding of health care need and delivery does the view emerge that providing chronic pain management is a choice? How can withdrawing treatment of childhood pain be thought to be morally acceptable?

We should remember that there is a small minority of patients who will gain access to appropriate care, including to residential treatment programs. However, the harsh and ugly reality is that the majority of adolescents with chronic pain and disability will go untreated, and unfortunately, many may live unhappily ever after.

In this chapter we have argued that there is an evidence base to support multidisciplinary chronic pain management for adolescents with chronic pain. However, there is no evidence to suggest that one model of care is more effective than any other model of care. Also, there is no evidence to support a public health solution to the problem of chronic pain. Therefore, local solutions with international lessons are necessary to drive change. In the absence of evidence, we here attempt to distill guidance that can provide a framework for the development of a model of treatment.

1. Establish need. What data are available to judge need or demand for services? Included in this are hidden and misdiagnosed needs.
2. Differentiate need and define a language for subpopulations of patients (e.g., complex disability and chronic pain or complex chronic pain).
3. Establish the costs of untreated pain and disability, both human and financial. This includes the costs of untreated pain that lie in other department's budgets.
4. Develop an understanding of the host organization. It is important to know the values of the organization and the models of care that the organization has experience delivering. It is important to establish whether the host organization is likely to understand chronic care.
5. Establish and actively manage stakeholders in untreated pain.
6. Decide which environmental features are essential to the model of delivery and which environmental features can be used within the delivery of the treatment.
7. Establish the model of treatment and evidence for the active agents of treatment.
8. Establish auditable outcomes in the language of each of the main stakeholders.
9. Accept that the delivery of adolescent chronic pain management will require all staff to develop a moral and political position on the importance of treatment.

We believe that there is evidence for the effectiveness of residential treatment programs for chronic pain in adolescents. There are health benefits that can obtain from the sojourn away from normal environments to gain access to a well-defined program of therapy. Simple absence from home is unlikely to have health benefits for the patient. What matters is that the reasons for the residential nature of a treatment have been made explicit, are internally consistent, and can be justified to the different stakeholders.

12. "Inconclusion"

Endings are also beginnings. If you look carefully at our fading tale, then you will see our noble queen emerging out of the mists that surround the Forest of Bureaucracy, from where few have returned alive. In the dead of night, she purloined a cloak from one of the riders of health care reality and infiltrated their camp. Although at first she found it to be a foreign and terrifying land where there was only the brutish barking of commands and a babble of anxious voices talking at once about a seemingly omnipresent specter, which she could just make out to be a demon they called rising costs, she came to learn that not all was lost, that there was hope.

She found no enemy, no dragon to be slain. Instead, what she found were yet more subjects in need of a common language and a common purpose. On her return to her beloved land, she ordered her barons to research and develop a common currency of need, to engage all of her people, whatever their health care creed, in a debate about common principles, common values, and a common willingness to treat, or to accept as untreated, chronic pain and suffering.

References

1. Perquin CW, Hazebroek-Kampscheur AAJM, Hunfeld JAM, et al. Pain in children and adolescents: a common experience. Pain 2000;87:51–58.
2. Fearon I, McGrath PJ, Achat H. "Booboos": the study of everyday pain among young children. Pain 1996;68:55–62.
3. Perquin CW, Hazebroek-Kampscheur AAJM, Hunfeld JAM, van Suijlekom-Smit LWA, Passchier J, van der Wouden JC. Chronic pain among children and adolescents: physician consultation and medication use. Clin J Pain 2001;16: 229–235.
4. Morris JN, Hardman AE. Walking to health. Sports Med 1997;23:306–332.
5. Kristjansdottir G, Rhee H. Risk factors of back pain frequency in schoolchildren: a search for explanations to a public health problem. Acta Paediatr 2002;91:849–854.
6. Mackenzie WG, Sampath JS, Kruse RW, Sheir Neiss GJ. Backpacks in children. Clin Orthop 2003:409:78–84.
7. Watson KD, Papageorgiou AC, Jones GT, et al. Low back pain in schoolchildren: the role of mechanical and psychosocial factors. Arch Dis Child 2003:88:12–17.
8. Wedderkopp N, Leboeuf-Yde C, Andersen LB, Froberg K, Hansen HS. Back pain in children. No association with objectively measured level of physical activity. Spine 2003;28:2019–2024.
9. Feldman DE, Barnett T, Shrier I, Rossignol M, Abenhaim L. Is physical activity differentially associated with different types of sedentary pursuits? Arch Pediatr Adolesc Med 2003;157:797–802.
10. Steig RL, Shepard TA. Pain medicine, the insurance industry, and health care reform. In: Cohen MJM, Campbell JN, eds., Pain Treatment Centers at a Crossroads: a Practical and Conceptual Reappraisal. Seattle, WA: IASP Press; 1996.

11. Cohen MJM. The pain center: centerpiece of comprehensive medicine? In: Cohen MJM, Campbell JN, eds., Pain Treatment Centers at a Crossroads: a Practical and Conceptual Reappraisal. Seattle, WA: IASP Press; 1996.

12. Wakai S, Ito N, Adachi N, Ueda D, Tsutsumi H, Chiba S. Hospice care for children. Lancet 1996;348:1102.

13. Mann T. The Magic Mountain. London: Penguin Books; 1924.

14. Murakami H. Norwegian Wood. London: Vintage Press; 1987.

15. Corr CA, Corr DM. Children's hospice care. Death Stud 1992;16:431–449.

16. Davies B. Assessment of need for a children's hospice program. Death Stud 1996;20:247–268.

17. Davies B, Collins J, Steele R, Pipke N, Cook K. Impact on families of a children's hospice program: evaluation. J Palliat Care 2000;16:63.

18. Franks PJ, Salisbury C, Bosanquet N, et al. The level of need for palliative care: a systematic review of the literature. Palliat Med 2000;14:93–104.

19. Mahoney JL, Schweder AE, Stattin H. Structured after-school activities as a moderator of depressed mood for adolescents with detached relations to their parents. J Community Psychol 2002;30:69–86.

20. Culp RH. Adolescent girls and outdoor recreation: a case study examining constraints and effective programming. J Leis Res 1998;30:356–379.

21. Plante WA, Lobato D, Engel R. Review of group interventions for pediatric chronic conditions. J Pediatr Psychol 2001;26:435–453.

22. Kiernan G, Gormly M, MacLachlan M. Outcomes associated with participation in a therapeutic recreation camping programme for children from 15 European countries: data from the "Barretstown Studies." Soc Sci Med 2004;903–913.

23. Suris J-C, Michaud P-A, Viner R. The adolescent with a chronic condition. Part I: development issues. Arch Dis Child 2004;89:938–942.

24. Michaud P-A, Suirs J-C, Viner R. The adolescent with a chronic condition. Part II: healthcare provision. Arch Dis Child 2004;89:943–949.

25. Jones R, Finlay F, Kreitman T. How can adolescent's health needs and concerns best be met? Br J Gen Pract 1997;47:631–634.

26. Suresh S, Doull IJM, Thomas P. Adolescent inpatient units. Arch Dis Child 2000; 82:266.

27. Sherry DD, Wallace CA, Kelley C, Kidder M, Sapp L. Short- and long-term outcomes of children with complex regional pain syndrome type I treated with exercise therapy. Clin J Pain 1999;15:218–223.

28. Malleson PN, Connell H, Bennett S, Eccleston C. Chronic idiopathic pain syndromes. Arch Dis Child 2001;84:193–199.

29. Sherry DD, Malleson PN. The idiopathic musculoskeletal pain syndromes in childhood. Rheum Dis Clin North Am 2002;28:669–685.

30. Eccleston C, Malleson PM. Management of chronic pain in children and adolescents [editorial]. BMJ 2003;326:1408, 1409.

31. Rolls R. The Hospital of the Nation: the Story of Spa Medicine and the Mineral Water Hospital at Bath. Bath, UK: BIRD Press; 1988.

32. McCracken L, Vowles K, Eccleston C. Acceptance-based treatment for persons with complex, long standing chronic pain: a preliminary analysis of treatment outcome in comparison to a waiting phase. Behav Res Ther 2005;43:1335–1346.

33. Eccleston Z, Eccleston C. Interdisciplinary management of adolescent chronic pain: developing the role of the physiotherapist. Physiotherapy 2004;90:77–81.

34. Stallard P. Think Good-Feel Good: a Cognitive Behaviour Therapy Workbook for Children and Young People. London: Wiley; 2002.

35. Hayes SC, Strosahl K, Wilson KG. Acceptance and Commitment Therapy: an Experiential Approach to Behavior Change. New York: Guildford; 1999.

36. McCracken LM, Carson JW, Eccleston C, Keefe FJ. Acceptance and change in the context of chronic pain. Pain 2004;109:4–7.

37. McCracken LM. Contextual Cognitive Behaviour Therapy for Chronic Pain. Seattle, WA: IASP Press, 2005.

38. Kabat-Zinn J, Lipworth L, Burney R. The clinical use of mindfulness meditation for the self-regulation of chronic pain. J Behav Med 1985;8;163–190.

39. Bishop SR, Lau M, Shapiro S, et al. Mindfulness: a proposed operational definition. Clin Psychol 2004;11:230–241.

40. Eccleston C, Morley S, Williams A, Yorke L, Mastroyannopoulou A. Systematic review and a subset meta-analysis of randomised controlled trials of psychological therapy for children and adolescents with chronic pain. Pain 2002;99:157–165.

41. Eccleston C, Malleson PM, Clinch J, Connell H, Sourbut C. Chronic pain in adolescents: evaluation of a programme of inter-disciplinary cognitive behaviour therapy (ICBT). Arch Dis Child 2003;88:881–885.

42. Eccleston C, Crombez G, Scotford A, Clinch J, Connell H. Adolescent chronic pain: patterns and predictors of emotional distress in adolescents with chronic pain and their parents. Pain 2004;108:221–229.

43. Morley S, Eccleston C, Williams A. Systematic review of cognitive behavioural therapy for the treatment of adult chronic pain. Pain 1999;80:1–13.

44. Fonagy P, Target M, Cottrell D, Phillips J, Kurtz Z. What Works for Whom? A Critical Review of Treatments for Children and Adolescents. London: Guildford Press; 2002.

45. Carter A. The Bloody Chamber. London: Penguin Books; 1979.

5

Managing Pediatric Pain at School

Ronald T. Brown

Summary

This chapter reviews literature pertaining to the management of pain within the school setting. Etiological issues underlying obstacles to school attendance are reviewed, including issues pertaining to make-up work, concerns among many children pertaining to use of the bathroom at school, diet and eating habits at school, relationship with a teacher or peer, fear of pain episodes at school, learning problems, test or performance anxiety, separation anxiety, and familial reinforcement of sick behavior. Interventions to increase school attendance are reviewed; these also include a careful assessment of the child and the family system, the use of behavioral interventions, as well as other treatment approaches, including the use of relaxation therapy and problem-solving therapy. Finally, specific directions for future research efforts and training also are provided.

Key Words: Anxiety; pain; pediatric; recurrent abdominal pain; school.

1. School as a Venue for Health Care

Reforms in health care have resulted in increased emphasis on specific access to care and the reduction of costs. One of the pathways of shifting health-related services is from tertiary care centers to primary care and community settings *(1)*. Because existing mechanisms in schools can serve children and adolescents with special needs, schools have been identified as a viable option for placement of community health care services. As Power and colleagues observed, schools are uniquely positioned to assist in the management and prevention of children's health problems *(2)*.

Several other factors support the change in focus of health care delivery from tertiary care settings to community settings *(1)*. These include advances in child development that underscore a social–ecological model by attending to all systems in the child's life (e.g., home, school). Moreover, the limitations of the medical model that traditionally has assumed a deficit model in health care have

From: *Bringing Pain Relief to Children: Treatment Approaches*
Edited by: G. A. Finley, P. J. McGrath, and C. T. Chambers © Humana Press Inc., Totowa, NJ

become increasingly apparent. Prevention, resilience, and positive adaptation have become the mainstays in health care. In support of this change, a number of interventions use elementary schools to address prevention of injury, including playground safety, seatbelt safety, fire safety, avoidance of spinal cord injuries, home safety programs, child sexual abuse programs, drug abuse education, driver education, and school violence *(3)*.

School interventions offer opportunities like easy access to assessment data, a venue to examine specific functions of behavior, the possibility of multidisciplinary teams for collaboration on assessment and remedy of specific behavior, and access to multiple change agents (e.g., peers, teachers) *(1)*. School personnel are ideally positioned for intervening directly in the child's natural environment, monitoring interventions in this environment, and providing a context for observing how competent, healthy children develop.

As noted, the social–ecological model underscores the importance of integrating systems of care, including the school. Child competencies and behaviors are observed not only at home but also at school. For example, a child with sickle cell disease will show specific symptoms or functional impairments at home and school. Thus, the school is an excellent place to assess impairments and implement intervention efforts. Stressors associated with a disease (e.g., the numerous painful events associated with sickle cell) are frequently manifested at school (e.g., problems with achievement or peer relationships). For disorders with recurrent pain, the stress that occurs at school will likely have an impact on functioning and decrease performance.

As Walker observed, life stress may play an especially crucial role in either precipitating or sustaining pain symptoms *(4)*. For example, Walker and associates noted that children with recurrent abdominal pain reported a greater frequency of daily stressors relative to their healthy peers *(5)*. Such stressors were associated with school-related activities, and disease included difficulty in comprehending homework assignments and excessive worries about examinations and grades. Children with recurrent abdominal pain also reported excessive anxiety and dysthymia on days that they also experienced stressful events. Walker and colleagues observed that these children reacted to stressful events with abdominal pain and other somatic symptoms, and the researchers concluded that children with recurrent pain may have a specific type of stress reactivity that manifests itself with specific somatic symptoms. Whether this is true for children with all types of recurrent pain is unclear. However, the role of stress and how to cope with stress are clearly associated with successful pain management.

Tsao and colleagues examined associations between gender and laboratory pain reactivity to the cold pressor task, a laboratory-placed analog that most closely approximates real pain experiences *(6)*. School absences and self-initiated school nurse visits were also examined in 57 children ranging in age from 8 to 10 years. Cold pressor task pain ratings, tolerance to pain, and gender were examined in relation to nurse visits and school absences. The number of nurse visits and school absences were collected over 2 years. Higher pain ratings and female sex predicted more school absences. In addition, female sex also predicted more frequent nurse visits for acute complaints with documented physical findings. Moreover, data suggested that girls are more likely than boys to miss school and visit the nurse for acute illnesses. These findings are important because they suggest the potential for screening children who may be especially vulnerable to frequent school absences based on self-reports of pain. The results from this investigation also indicate that girls may be especially vulnerable to functional impairments (i.e., school attendance) because of recurrent pain.

In a follow-up study to the Tsao et al. investigation *(6)*, Tsao and Zeltzer examined sex differences in self-initiated school nurse visits and pain-associated symptoms in 57 preadolescents aged 9–11 years *(7)*. The preadolescents were asked to complete the pain-focused version of the Children's Somatization Inventory. Pain symptom scores, gender, and the interaction of pain symptoms and gender were examined in relationship to nurse visits that were tracked over 1 year. Neither sex nor pain scores alone predicted total nurse visits. For female preadolescents, higher pain symptom scores predicted total visits for complaints with documented physical findings. This was consistent with the findings of the elementary school sample conducted by Tsao et al. *(6)*. A complex association was demonstrated in this preadolescent sample among gender, pain-related symptoms, and self-initiated nurse visits. Again, the investigators interpreted their data to suggest that pain-focused symptom measures may predict later pain management.

Tsao and Zeltzer suggested that the identification of these symptoms by self-report measures may be important in predicting health care utilization, particularly for young adults *(7)*. Whether preadolescent pain management or adolescent pain management predicts later coping with pain during young adulthood is an important area of inquiry for future research. Clearly, longitudinal studies will be needed in this area, particularly studies using longitudinal methodology.

Walker and Greene demonstrated that children who experience a number of negative life events are more apt to exhibit pain symptoms over time relative to children reporting few negative life events *(8)*. The researchers hypothesized that these children have difficulty deriving support from others, particularly peers, because they also are involved in fewer peer activities relative to their healthy peers. Walker suggested that interventions designed to assist children and adolescents in increasing social competencies with peers may concomitantly enhance these children's capacity to cope with pain symptoms *(4)*.

In support of the notion that negative life events or the absence of peer social support may be associated with frequent health symptoms, Williams and coworkers estimated the prevalence of bullying in nearly 3000 elementary schoolchildren in a large urban area in the United Kingdom *(9)*. The investigators examined the association of bullying with common health symptoms in childhood. The dependent measures in the investigation included self-reported bullying and common health symptoms. Approximately one-fourth of the cohort for whom information was available reported that they had been bullied. An association was found between children who reported being bullied and not sleeping well, bed wetting, symptoms of depression, and experiences of minor somatic symptoms, including headaches and stomachaches. There was a positive association between increasing risk of health symptoms and bullying. These data provide compelling evidence for the association between somatic symptoms and peer supports. The investigators cautioned that this association may not necessarily be causal, but they underscored the role of peer support in children's coping with somatic issues. Studies are needed that systematically examine objective measures of peer relationships, including peer sociometry as rated by other peers and the relationship of these assessments to somatic symptoms and coping with pain.

As Walker cautioned, most investigations of children with recurrent pain have been conducted on pediatric patients in tertiary care facilities *(4)*. The pain of these children is likely to be of longer duration and is more likely to be accompanied by significant psychiatric comorbidity, as well as be refractory to traditional treatments, relative to children evaluated and treated in a primary care facility. Walker observed that distress among these patients may be higher than in community or school samples, suggesting that problems identified in the primary care office or school setting may also be identified rather easily and readily managed by caregivers and school professionals. Epidemiological studies are needed that systematically examine potential differences between children and adolescents who are brought to their primary care providers vs children who come to a tertiary care setting.

2. Obstacles to School Attendance

Walker delineated several obstacles to school attendance *(4)*. These include problems with make-up work, explanations to teachers and peers regarding why the children may have missed so many days of school, children's reluctance to use bathrooms at their schools, diet and eating habits at school, relationship with a teacher or peers, fear of pain episodes at school, learning problems, test or performance anxiety, separation anxiety, and family reinforcement of sick role behavior. Walker noted that a gradual return may help children return to school full time. Such a schedule may also assist them in eventually regaining their confidence that they can survive a pain episode at school. Walker suggested that full-time attendance is typically possible within 3–4 weeks after the implementation of a program designed to help school attendance for children with pain episodes.

2.1. Make-Up Work

Many children seem to be overwhelmed by the amount of make-up work when they return to school after a prolonged illness *(4)*. Some children fear that they may not be able to complete all of the work, or that they may not understand the assignments. These feelings of self-doubt and negative cognitions may even exacerbate pain symptoms. In these cases, Walker suggested a structured plan in which a missed assignment is broken into manageable parts, with a schedule that underscores specific progress toward accomplishing missed assignments rather than completing final products. Caregivers and teachers can establish specific periods of time for making up missed assignments (e.g., performing make-up work for approx 30 minutes/day). Frequently, caregivers must contact the school to determine what make-up work will be required and to negotiate a reasonable timeline for completing the assignments. A reduction in work assignments will sometimes be necessary if the child cannot manage the completion of the tasks within a specific time frame.

2.2. Explanations to Teachers and Peers

Many children become anxious that teachers or peers may ask them why they have been absent from school, particularly if the illness does not have a specific organic etiology or medical tests may not be conclusive in identifying specific pathology. As Walker suggested, some children may need specific assistance in preparing a response *(4)*. In other cases, it may be helpful to have a letter from the child's primary care provider indicating that the illness is legitimate. The primary care provider could recommend returning to school for only part of the day or using the bathroom whenever the child deems it necessary. Walker et al. acknowledged that, even in the absence of any identifiable organic disease, pain may be as severe and functionally incapacitating as in conditions for which there is identifiable organic pain *(10)*. It is important that professionals communicate an acknowledgment of pain and clarify coping strategies in pain management *(4)*.

2.3. School Bathrooms

Many children with gastrointestinal disorders or recurrent abdominal pain may be reluctant to use the bathrooms at their school *(4)*. These children may avoid school bathrooms because of lack of privacy, poor sanitation, lack of toilet paper, or the fear that classmates may know that they are defecating in the bathroom. In some cases, children may fear either physical or verbal abuse by other children while in the bathroom. In other cases, children may fear that using the bathroom may take too long and could eventually result in reprimands from the teacher for tardiness. Walker suggested the health care provider write a letter to the school indicating that the child should be allowed to use the bathroom whenever necessary. This would put the timing of bathroom use under the child's control and diminish anxiety about accidents. In addition, it will allow the child to use the bathroom when peers are not present. Parents can advocate for sanitary bathroom facilities in the public schools. Walker also suggested that children learn to use public bathrooms in specific progressive stages, beginning with bathrooms in the homes of friends and relatives and subsequently restaurants and private buildings. The child can be rewarded for using bathroom facilities in new settings, which it is hoped will generalize to school settings and enhance self-competence and adaptation to pain experiences outside the home.

2.4. Diet and Eating Habits at School

For children with recurrent abdominal pain, Walker noted that diet and eating habits may exacerbate symptoms *(4)*. Available foods and schedules for school lunch may contribute to symptoms. Many children may not have sufficient time to ingest their food and use the bathroom in the amount of time provided for lunch. In other cases, the types of food and beverages may also increase gastrointestinal symptoms and result in abdominal distress. In such cases, parents can advocate for specialized diets. With the epidemic of obesity in children and adolescents and the resulting increased risk for other diseases (e.g., type 2 diabetes, cardiovascular problems), it would be appropriate for the school to advocate for good nutritional standards in promoting positive health behaviors.

2.5. Relationship With a Teacher or Peer

In many cases, children with recurrent pain, particularly recurrent abdominal pain, may have difficulty adjusting to a teacher who is more matter-of-fact or less nurturing than previous teachers, which is sometimes misinterpreted by some children as disapproval *(4,11)*. In such cases, it is useful for the parents to meet with the teacher, principal, or school counselor to get to know the teacher better. In many cases, after frank discussion, the teacher can assist in helping the child to adjust, and the child can better understand the teacher's style.

As Walker asserted, a change of teachers should only be initiated as a last resort *(4)*. Such a change could reinforce beliefs or distortions that the child is unable to cope with. Also, additional stressors might result in adjusting to a new classroom, particularly for a child who already has other stressors and perhaps inadequate coping skills. Some children report taunting or teasing by peers in the classroom. In such cases, it is useful for caregivers to meet with school personnel to work jointly in resolving such issues.

2.6. Fear of Pain Episodes at School

Children who have poor coping skills for dealing with pain may often harbor exaggerated fears that they will have a pain episode at school and not be able to manage it. Walker observed that such distress arises from an ongoing habit of focusing attention on minor physical sensations and fearing these sensations will increase in intensity *(4)*. This results in noxious sensory experiences, increased anticipatory pain, increased anxiety, physiological arousal, diminished pain thresholds, and increased distress *(12,13)*. This is a cyclical effect in which anxiety about pain diminishes pain thresholds and capacity for coping with pain.

A primary goal in working with these children is to assist them in learning that they can cope with their pain *(4)*. Walker recommended that children's initial return to school be brief, perhaps only 1–2 hours/day. Most children will be able to attend school and even manage their pain for brief periods. The brief school attendance will assist children in building confidence so they may later be able to survive a pain episode at school. The child's health care provider and caregivers should have a plan in place in case the child experiences pain while at school. It is typically best if the child is allowed to lie down and rest until well enough to return to class or until it is time to leave school for the day. A child may also work with a school counselor to learn relaxation or distraction techniques *(4,14)*. Walker cautioned it is often counterproductive for children to call home or be allowed to leave school early when a pain episode occurs as this reinforces complaining and passive coping styles. Walker et al. noted that children who use passive coping strategies like withdrawal (e.g., remaining home from school or returning home quickly after attending school for a short period of time) are more likely to maintain these patterns and symptoms over the long term *(5)*.

2.7. Learning Problems

A history of academic difficulties in one or more subject areas, problems with attention and concentration, failure to complete assignments, or an inappropriate class placement may signify a learning problem or a stressful experience. Some children may use pain to cope with such difficulties. To increase coping skills, caregivers may need to contact school personnel to develop a plan that might include special education services, tutoring, or assistance with organizational skills *(4)*. Efforts should be made to minimize the chance of the plan failing, and procedures should be implemented that allow the child to make a smooth transition back to school.

2.8. Test or Performance Anxiety

Many children report a greater frequency of pain symptoms prior to a stressful event or competitive activity at school, including athletic events and examinations *(4)*. Such circumscribed anxiety may benefit from the use of positive self-coaching statements, such as, "I know I can do it if I just do my best." Negative self-statements, such as "What if I fail?," should be eliminated. The use of adaptive self-statements is important to enhance coping strategies and diminish distorted negative thoughts when approaching stressful tasks.

2.9. Separation Anxiety

Separation anxiety refers to developmentally inappropriate and excessive anxiety concerning separation from home or from those to whom the child is attached *(15)*. One symptom criterion for the diagnosis of separation anxiety disorder includes "repeated complaints of physical symptoms (such as headaches or stomachaches, nausea or vomiting) when separation from major attachment figures occurs or is anticipated" (p. 113). Typically, such symptoms occur on the morning of schooldays and are less pervasive on weekends when the child will not be separated from caregivers *(4)*. Symptoms may reoccur on Sunday evening in anticipation of separation from caregivers to attend school on Monday.

Other symptoms of separation anxiety include recurrent or excessive distress when separation from home or major attachment figures occurs or is anticipated; persistent and excessive worry about losing, or possible harm befalling, major attachment figures; persistent and excessive worry that an untoward event will lead to separation from a major attachment figure (e.g., getting lost or being kidnapped). Other issues include persistent reluctance or refusal to go to school or elsewhere because of fear of separation, persistent and excessive fearfulness or reluctance to be alone without major attachment figures at home or without significant adults in other settings, persistent reluctance or refusal to go to sleep without being near a major attachment figure or to sleep away from home, and repeated nightmares involving the theme of separation *(15)*.

In accordance with psychiatric criteria, the duration of disturbance must be at least 4 weeks, and the onset must before age 18 *(15)*. There must also be some functional impairment, including clinically significant distress or impairment in social, academic, or other important areas of functioning. In addition, separation anxiety disorder does not occur exclusively during the course of a pervasive developmental disorder, schizophrenia, or other psychotic disorder and, in adolescents and adults, is not better accounted for by panic disorder with agoraphobia.

Often, caregivers of children with separation anxiety disorder have an enmeshed relationship with their children. Children may sleep with their parents and may sit very close to the parents during the interview *(4)*. Both the caregiver and the child tend to perceive pain as so severe that it makes school attendance impossible. Because a complete cure for many types of pain is quite difficult to accomplish, caregivers must be convinced that it is necessary to teach their children appropriate coping skills for managing pain. It is important for caregivers to support their children in attending school for at least part of the day despite their children's pain. A primary goal of treatment is to thwart the cycle of the separation anxiety for both the caregivers and the child. Thus, it is recommended that caregivers and their children be allowed initially to limit attendance at school for a specific amount of time so they can be confident of their success in managing pain at school. This period of time will vary depending on the severity of separation anxiety. School attendance must be reinforced by the caregiver, so it is necessary for the caregiver to be comfortable with the child's partial return to school.

2.10. Family Reinforcement of Sick Behavior

No specific differences have been found between families of well children and those of children with chronic pain on family measures like marital satisfaction and cohesion *(4)*. However, some clinical evidence suggests that these families may differ in areas not gaged by standardized instruments. Overprotectiveness and enmeshment are two of these areas. Walker suggested that social modeling of pain may contribute to recurrent pain episodes among children, particularly if the child vicariously observes a parent receiving attention from other family members if there are complaints of pain. Levy and coworkers noted that a child may learn pain behavior when caregivers seek extensive medical consultation for pain *(16)*. Walker noted that caregivers of children with abdominal pain may view their children as vulnerable, and these caregivers may attempt to protect their children from potential health-related threats *(4)*. This pattern may result in caregivers letting a child stay home from school because of minor ailments like stomachaches.

Walker et al. noted that absences from school may serve to reinforce a child's pain behavior, particularly when the child is excused from examinations, sporting events, or other activities that involve performance *(17)*. This is especially true for children who fear failure. In addition, the researchers observed that some children may gain social reinforcement (i.e., special attention, privileges) as a result of their symptoms, which in turn may increase sick role behaviors. Walker et al. reported that children with recurrent abdominal pain perceived their caregivers as providing them with greater attention and relief from responsibilities than that reported by other children *(10)*.

Thus, children may gain special attention for sick behavior or their illness. In these cases, it is useful to have specific guidelines (e.g., fever) for caregivers regarding when children should be allowed to remain home from school. The child who stays home should be made to remain in bed during the day, eliminating reinforcement of sick role behaviors *(4)*. It is also wise for schools to provide reinforcement for behaviors that are associated with competence, such as school attendance.

2.11. Summary

For children with chronic pain, there are a number of common obstacles to school attendance that must be assessed before implementing any treatment program designed to increase school attendance *(4,18)*. These obstacles include children being overwhelmed by make-up work, concerns about explanations to teachers and peers about the pain, concern about the use of school bathrooms, particularly for children and adolescents with recurrent abdominal pain, problems with relationships with teachers and peers, fear of painful episodes at school, presence of learning problems or inappropriate school or classroom placement, test performance or anxiety, separation anxiety, the family's reinforcement of the child's sick role behavior, children's emotional distress, and general life stress. It is imperative that the practitioners evaluate these issues before designing or implementing a plan or program for the child to return to school.

3. Increasing School Attendance

3.1. Assessment

The most important step in assisting children's return to school is the identification of specific obstacles to school attendance *(4,18)*. The pediatric or mental health provider must conduct a detailed assessment of obstacles to school attendance. Questions about obstacles to school attendance should be nonthreatening and designed to solicit general conversation with the child about school. Typically, conversations with children will provide a great deal of information about school attendance and issues of anxiety. In general, this is a time for the provider to establish rapport with the child. In most cases, it is usually not helpful to ask yes or no questions because open-ended questions will elicit more from the child.

Walker constructed a specific semistructured interview for providers *(4)*. Questions might include the following: What do you like best (least) about school? Which grade do you like better, the one you are in now or the grade you were in last year? What was your favorite year (favorite teacher) in school? Why? What is similar or different about this school year? What will it be like when you go back to school? Do you have a lot of make-up work? What will the kids (teacher) say when they see you? Will the teacher be glad to see you? What will you do if you have a stomachache (or other pain) at school? Will you be able to use the bathroom at school when you need to? Do you sleep in your own room at night? Does anyone sleep with you? How do you spend the day when you stay home from school?

Responses to these questions will provide information to the practitioner about obstacles to school attendance and identification of specific stressors surrounding school attendance. After determining the stressors, the provider can work with the family and school personnel for interventions that improve school attendance. It is especially important to work with children on school-related issues in anticipation of future medical regimens, coping with returning to school, managing peer questions, or concerns about disfigurement (e.g., in the case of burns).

A careful analysis is critical in the identification of factors that may contribute to the child's or the family's reluctance about the child's return to school. These data should be elicited from both the child and the caregiver in a forthright interview, with specific questions about coping with return to school, managing peer questions, and concerns about a new school environment.

3.2. Interventions

Walker recommended that a graduated plan be implemented that incorporates as its ultimate optimal goal returning to school full time *(4)*. This is suggested because some children, particularly those who have separation anxiety, will become distressed at any mention of returning to school. Walker acknowledged that, if children with recurrent pain are required to attend school the day following their medical evaluation, it is likely that they may manifest a severe pain episode that will serve to prevent or impede school attendance. As noted, an important first step in assisting children in their return to school is the identification of obstacles and addressing these specific issues and concerns *(4,18)*. Walker also suggested that the health care provider consult with both the child and the caregiver to identify a manageable goal for initial attendance at school. The provider generally begins with the goal of a half-day return to school. If the child or caregiver notes concern, the time might be decreased until both the child and caregiver are confident that the child will be able to succeed.

In developing any type of intervention program, the health care provider should contract the child's caregivers to determine their motivation. Also, caregivers need to acknowledge they will be amenable to obtaining additional assistance if the child is not successful in the treatment program *(4)*. Typically, a child should be successful in returning to school at least within 3 weeks after commencement of the program.

3.2.1. Behavioral Approaches

It is recommended that a program be implemented that reinforces school attendance. Such an approach might include a token economy system in which the child receives ongoing reinforcement for progress in attending school. For example, the use of small incremental periods of school attendance might be reinforced with either special privileges or small rewards. Points might be earned and eventually traded for larger prizes. As Walker noted, it is important to consider the specific characteristics of the child and the family and to use a reward system that is sufficiently reinforcing to the child *(4)*. Also, make sure the family is capable of implementing the system. It is critical that returning to school be a family affair, with all family members in agreement on the contingencies and the reinforcers. The family must be sufficiently organized to apply the reinforcement in a timely and consistent manner immediately after the desired behavior of school attendance is achieved. The system of rewards should be motivating enough that the child is interested in receiving additional rewards, and full school attendance will eventually be possible. The rewards may be increased or decreased on a variable schedule. Additional reinforcers may also be provided to increase other desired behaviors (e.g., not crying when returning to school). Verbal praise should always be provided in addition to tangible rewards. Further, as children lose interest in the current rewards, a system should be in place for new rewards that are meaningful and desirable for the child and will also motivate desired behavior.

Ultimately, a system might be used in which the child could trade points for larger rewards over a longer period of time. Eventually, longer-term goals can replace shorter-term goals until the eventual goal of returning to school full time is accomplished. For issues of separation anxiety, children may have more difficulty in separating from one parent than another. In such situations, the parent from whom it is easier to detach should bring the child to school. Review the behavioral program on an ongoing basis to evaluate its efficacy and to develop additional long-term goals *(4)*.

3.2.2. Other Treatment Approaches

Other treatment approaches have been evaluated for children and adolescents with recurrent pain. These approaches have primarily involved relaxation training designed to diminish frequency and intensity of pain *(14,19,20)*. Larsson and Carlson discussed the advantages of treatment programs in schools for children and adolescents with chronic pain *(14)*. School health professionals (e.g., a school nurse, school psychologist) who are available to children during school hours and between training sessions can manage such programs. When such approaches are administered at school, they may be potentially offered in a group format, thereby serving as many children and adolescents in need as possible. Implementation of such programs at school enhances the possibility of external validity or generalizability. Such approaches are cost-effective and may be implemented by school personnel.

Larsson and Melin conducted an experimental study of 32 adolescent high school students who ranged in age from 16 to 18 years *(19)*. All of the adolescents were identified with various types of chronic headaches, including tension and combined tension and migraine headaches. All of the participants were treated in school. Participants were assigned randomly to a nine-session relaxation training program or to an information-contact condition. Both of these treatment conditions were contrasted to a no-contact control condition. Relaxation therapy alone resulted in the reduction of headache complaints. Participants at their 6-month follow-up evaluations continued to have fewer complaints. The effects obtained in the information-contact showed only minor improvements relative to the relaxation condition. Although this investigation did not lend itself to issues of separation anxiety or returning to school, the findings are important because they demonstrate the efficacy and success of a pain intervention program at school.

Larsson and associates conducted a controlled trial in which the efficacy of a self-help relaxation approach was compared with problem discussion and a self-monitoring condition *(20)*. Participants were 36 high school students who suffered from tension and combined tension and migraine headaches. The students were treated during a 5-week period in a traditional school system. The self-help relaxation treatment condition resulted in improvements on all dimensions of the participants' headaches. Conclusions from the investigation were that self-help relaxation training is a promising, cost-effective procedure to manage chronic headaches in adolescents. These investigators demonstrated the viability of such an intervention in a high school setting.

In a more recent investigation, Larsson and Carlsson compared the efficacy of a school-based, nurse-administered relaxation training intervention with a no-treatment control condition for 26 children and adolescents ranging in age from 10 to 15 years *(14)*. All of the participants in the investigation suffered from chronic tension headaches. Participants were assigned randomly to either the relaxation intervention or the no-treatment control group. They were assessed pre- and posttesting and at a 6-month follow-up. Headache activity for the children treated with relaxation training was significantly reduced relative to the control condition at both posttreatment and the 6-month follow-up. Specifically, 69 and 73% of the children and adolescents at posttest assessment and at 6-month follow-up, respectively, who were treated with relaxation had achieved clinically significant headache improvement (50% improvement) relative to 8% and 27% of the pupils in the control group, respectively. This investigation underscored the viability of such a treatment program in a school setting for children and adolescents with recurrent pain.

3.3. Summary

It is important to assess whether a family is organized, capable, and sufficiently motivated to implement a behavior management plan. A plan that emphasizes return to school on a graduated basis is generally most acceptable and effective, with the ultimate goal full return to school. Typically, such a plan takes approx 3 weeks to complete. If the child has not returned to school full time in the selected time, it is recommended that a mental health care provider be consulted for assistance. The initial goal for return to school should be made easy for the child and family to accomplish (e.g., returning to school for a portion of the day). Rewards for school attendance should be within the family's budget, and the rewards should be provided as soon as they are earned and not be available to the child by other means. Rewards can consist of small prizes, special activities, or stars that can be redeemed for other prizes or activities. The family also should be provided with a copy of the behavior plan reward schedule. The school should also be aware of the behavior plan for returning to school.

When rewards are given, parents should also provide verbal praise. Rewards should be given for each period of school attendance but should diminish over time as the behavior is more concretely in place. It is important that all caregivers be involved in the program, and that the program be reviewed on a regular basis for revision and to reflect accomplishments, new goals, and new rewards. Long-term goals should include sustained school attendance.

Few studies have examined interventions designed to manage recurrent pain in the school setting. There are a number of advantages to school-based interventions, including availability of personnel, access to many children, generalizability, and cost-effectiveness. The few studies that are available suggest the potential efficacy of these programs for managing recurrent headaches in the school setting. More clinical trials are needed and should involve the child, the school, and the family in management of recurrent pain.

4. Conclusions and Future Directions

Recurrent pain in children and adolescents represents a major public health concern. Concomitantly, numerous changes have permeated the delivery of health care services in the United States, including the provision of services at the level of primary care (21). The result has been a trend toward placing systems of care for pediatric populations into schools and a trend away from provision of services at the level of tertiary care centers. The school further represents a venue where additional disease prevention and health promotion can occur. Pain management may take place in schools, coping skills may be fostered, and partnerships may be forged among pediatricians, families, and mental health providers.

The importance of careful and ongoing assessment to identify potential barriers to school attendance must be underscored, particularly as these barriers are associated with recurrent pain episodes. Semistructured, structured, and paper-and-pencil self-report interview procedures should be used to identify barriers. Unfortunately, there is insufficient psychometric data on assessment techniques used in schools. The development and validation of assessment instruments are necessary, especially measurements designed to evaluate recurrent pain and how stressors associated with school attendance affect children's management and coping.

This chapter underscores the potential efficacy of behavioral approaches in supporting children's return to school. Numerous reasons for lack of school attendance are reviewed, including separation anxiety, fear of returning to school because of missed work, specific health- and pain-related issues that are made worse in the school setting, and inappropriate school placement. Despite the undisputed efficacy of behavioral approaches at school, potential barriers exist. These can include a lack of information among both caregivers and school professionals on the value of behavioral approaches. Other barriers that might impede implementation of these behavioral techniques include severe psychopathology of caregivers, lack of motivation on the part of caregivers and school personnel, and reinforcement systems that are not sufficiently motivating to the child or are not followed carefully.

Other therapeutic approaches like relaxation techniques and cognitive behavioral interventions given at school show promise. Such approaches may be applied to many children simultaneously. They are especially ecologically valid and generalizable and are cost-effective because they can be conducted by professionals already employed in the school system.

Much of what has been reviewed in this chapter points toward recommended changes in public policy for children who experience chronic pain and at the same time attend school. We anticipate that public policy ultimately will be expressed through federal and state legislation that it is hoped will dictate appropriate allocation of resources that allow for the incorporation of pediatric psychological and mental health services in schools. Many complex services will be needed for schools and the families served by them, including an increase in medical, educational, and psychological services. Perrin and Ireys observed that the organization of services for children with chronic illnesses is both diverse and fragmented *(22)*. A first effort and necessary first step will be to integrate pediatric and psychological services across multiple locations, including schools and pediatric health care settings.

Thompson and Gustafson underscored that a major source of stress in caring for children with chronic disease is economic *(23)*. Although efficiency in the provision of services is important, direct costs of services (e.g., mental health staff services, adjunctive care for families, and transportation for caregivers) will also be important. Legislation for specialized services to be provided to children and adolescents with recurrent and chronic pain can and should be advocated by the national associations representing pediatrics, psychology, and psychiatry.

Training efforts need to continue to focus on health care providers and the appropriate delivery of services in schools. Efforts need to be made to train school personnel, including school nurses and school psychologists, in the appropriate delivery of specialized pediatric psychological services in schools. Educational personnel also will need to be trained in the effect of chronic disease on the daily functioning of children, with a focus on academic achievement and successful socialization. Such training efforts will promulgate additional services for children and adolescents with recurrent pain and it is hoped will stimulate research by pain experts and pediatric and school psychologists. It is hoped that greater collaboration will provide better clinical services, long-needed research, and public policies that advocate for these children and their families.

References

1. Power TJ, Blom-Hoffman J. The school as a venue for managing and preventing health problems: opportunities and challenges. In: Brown RT, ed. Handbook of Pediatric Psychology in School Settings. Mahwah, NJ: Erlbaum; 2004, pp. 37–78.
2. Power TJ, Heathfield L, McGoey K, Blum NJ. Managing and preventing chronic health problems: school psychology's role. Sch Psychol Rev 1999;28:251–263.
3. Roberts MC, Brown KJ, Boles RE, Mashunkashey JO. Prevention of injuries: concepts and interventions for pediatric psychology in the schools. In: Brown RT, ed. Handbook of Pediatric Psychology in School Settings. Mahwah, NJ: Erlbaum; 2004, 65–80.
4. Walker LS. Helping the child with recurrent abdominal pain return to school. Pediatr Ann 2004;33:128–136.
5. Walker LS, Smith CA, Garber J, Van Slyke DA, Claar RL. The relation of daily stressors to somatic and emotional symptoms in children with and without recurrent abdominal pain. J Consult Clin Psychol 2001;69:85–91.
6. Tsao JCI, Glover DA, Bursch R, Ifewunigwe M, Zeltzer LK. Laboratory pain reactivity and gender: relationship to school nurse visits and school absences. J Dev Behav Pediatr 2002;23:217–224.
7. Tsao JC, Zeltzer LK. Sex differences in pain-related symptoms and self-initiated school nurse visits among pre-adolescents. J Pain Symptom Manage 2003;25: 472–480.
8. Walker LS, Greene JW. Negative life events and symptom resolution in pediatric abdominal pain patients. J Pediatr Psychol 1991;16:341–360.
9. Williams K, Chambers M, Logan S, Robinson D. Association of common health symptoms with bullying in primary school children. Br Med J 1996;313:17–19.

10. Walker LS, Garber J, Greene JW. Psychosocial characteristics of recurrent childhood pain: a comparison of children with recurrent abdominal pain, organic illness, and psychiatric disorders. J Abnorm Child Psychol 1993;102:248–258.

11. Claar RL, Walker LS. Maternal attributions for the causes and remedies of their children's abdominal pain. J Pediatr Psychol 1999;24:345–354.

12. Walker LS. The evolution of research on recurrent abdominal pain: history, assumptions, and a conceptual model. In: McGrath PJ, Finley GA, eds. Progress in Pain Research and Management. Vol. 13. Seattle, WA: IASP Press; 1999:141–172.

13. Zeltzer LK, Bush JP, Chen E, Riveral A. A psychobiologic approach to pediatric pain: part I. History, physiology, and assessment strategies. Curr Prob Pediatr 1997;27:255–258.

14. Larsson B, Carlson J. A school-based, nurse-administered relaxation training for children with chronic tension-type headache. J Pediatr Psychol 1996;21:603–614.

15. American Psychiatric Association. Diagnostic and Statistical Manual of Mental Disorders. 4th ed. Washington, DC: American Psychiatric Association; 1994.

16. Levy RL, Whitehead WE, Van Korff MR, Feld AD. Intergenerational transmission of gastrointestinal illness behavior. Am J Gastroenterol 2000;95:451–456.

17. Walker LS, Claar RL, Garber J. Social consequences of children's pain: when do they encourage symptom maintenance? J Pediatr Psychol 2002;27:689–698.

18. Walker LS, Johnson WS. Recurrent abdominal pain and functional gastrointestinal disorders in the school setting. In: Brown RT, ed. Handbook of Pediatric Psychology in School Settings. Mahwah, NJ: Erlbaum; 2004, pp. 299–312.

19. Larsson B, Melin L. Chronic headaches in adolescents: treatment in a school setting with relaxation training as compared with information-contact and self-registration. Pain 1986;25:325–336.

20. Larrson B, Melin L, Lamminen M, Ulstedt F. A school-based treatment of chronic headaches in adolescents. J Pediatr Psychol 1987;12:553–566.

21. Brown RT. Introduction: changes in the provision of health care to children and adolescents. In: Brown RT, ed. Handbook of Pediatric Psychology in School Settings. Mahwah, NJ: Erlbaum; 2004, pp. 1–19.

22. Perrin JM, Ireys HT. The organization of service for chronically ill children and their families. Ped Clin North Am 1984;31:235–257.

23. Thompson RJ Jr, Gustafson KE, Hamlet KW, Spock A. Stress, coping, and family functioning in the psychological adjustment of mothers of children and adolescents with cystic fibrosis. J Pediatr Psychol 1992;17:573–585.

6

Efficacy of Complementary and Alternative Medicine Approaches for Pediatric Pain

State of the Science

Jennie C. I. Tsao, Marcia Meldrum, and Lonnie K. Zeltzer

Summary

Pain may be a major cause of physical and emotional distress in chronic pediatric conditions, including cancer, juvenile arthritis, and cystic fibrosis. Complementary and alternative medical (CAM) therapies have become important and frequently used modalities in treating children's pain. Yet, many practitioners have questioned whether there is sufficient evidence to support the efficacy and safety of CAM approaches for pain relief. This chapter aims to address these concerns by presenting a critical review of the available published evidence. We evaluated published studies testing CAM interventions for chronic or acute procedural pain; these study methodologies employed either controlled trials or multiple baseline studies. The evaluation criteria were developed by the American Psychological Association Division 12 Task Force on Promotion and Dissemination of Psychological Procedures to assess nonpharmacological therapies. Few of the CAM modalities qualify as empirically supported therapies under these rigorous criteria, although several met the standard for possibly efficacious or promising for pediatric pain. Our review of the published literature revealed a number of methodological flaws in existing studies. Clearly, more research on CAM therapies for children's pain is needed.

Key Words: Alternative medicine; children; complementary medicine; pain; pediatric pain.

1. Introduction and Epidemiology

Complementary and alternative medicine (CAM) is defined as those therapeutic interventions not widely established for use in conventional health care practice or incorporated into the standard medical curriculum *(1)*. Although reports suggested that use of CAM has increased substantially in pediatric health care *(2)*, estimates of CAM use for the treatment of children vary from

From: *Bringing Pain Relief to Children: Treatment Approaches*
Edited by: G. A. Finley, P. J. McGrath, and C. T. Chambers © Humana Press Inc., Totowa, NJ

a bare 2% *(3)* to 20–30% in some communities *(2,4)*. A single consistent estimate is not possible because of variances in published reports in the populations studied, methodology employed, and definition of CAM used.

A population-based study representative of the general population of children younger than 18 years in the United States estimated CAM use at only 1.8% (95% confidence interval, 1.3–2.3%) *(3)*. However, this study assessed only whether respondents consulted a CAM practitioner, and prior work has shown that nearly half of those who used CAM did so without consulting a practitioner *(1)*. Thus, it is likely that this particular study underestimated use of CAM in children in the United States *(5,6)*.

Chronic pain is among the main conditions for which CAM is used in the US adult population *(7–9)* according to several national studies of representative samples. Bausell and colleagues *(8)* reported that musculoskeletal disorders (e.g., osteoarthritis, back disorders, joint disorders) ranked among the top three categories of reasons precipitating a visit to a CAM practitioner by 5.1% of adults, with mental disorders at 6.6% and metabolic disorders at 5.5%. An earlier study found that the conditions for which adults reported highest rates of CAM use were neck (57%) and back (47.6%) pain problems *(9)*.

There have been no population-based studies describing reasons for CAM use in children; however, it is recognized that children with chronic conditions that may be not responsive to conventional treatments appear to have particularly high rates of CAM use *(10)*. Thus, rates of CAM use among pediatric patients with chronic conditions, such as cancer, rheumatoid arthritis, and cystic fibrosis, range from 30 to 70% *(11,12)*. In many of these conditions, pain is often a significant problem.

The increased interest in CAM modalities for pediatric pain has raised concerns about the safety and efficacy of these interventions. The many published case reports and uncontrolled investigations may offer important clues, but only rigorously designed and carefully executed controlled studies can provide the evidence to substantiate the safe and effective use of CAM treatments for pediatric pain.

The American Psychological Association Division 12 Task Force on Promotion and Dissemination of Psychological Procedures (referred to here as the 1995 Task Force) *(13,14)* has developed a useful and rigorous set of criteria for the evaluation of nondrug therapies. As described by Chambless and Hollon *(13)*, the task force outlined criteria for designations of possibly efficacious, efficacious, and efficacious and specific. A treatment modality may be considered *efficacious* if a minimum of two between-group experiments conducted by at least two independent research groups have shown that the intervention is superior to a no-treatment control, an alternative treatment, or a placebo or equivalent to a previously established treatment. However, to be judged *efficacious and specific*, at least two independent research groups must have conducted studies that controlled for nonspecific effects (e.g., increased attention) that showed the modality to be superior to placebo or a previously established treatment. A modality may be designated *possibly efficacious* if there is only one between-group study demonstrating its superiority to a no-treatment control, alternative treatment, or placebo, or equivalence to standard treatment.

All studies used as evidence of efficacy should (1) use a treatment manual or logical equivalent; (2) test all interventions in a clearly delineated population with specified inclusion criteria and treated for specific problems; (3) use reliable and valid outcome measures; and (4) apply appropriate data analyses. Treatments meeting all these criteria may be considered empirically supported therapies (ESTs).

Our aim in this chapter is to evaluate the empirical evidence for the efficacy of CAM approaches for pediatric pain using the task force guidelines. All CAM interventions reviewed are supported by existing literature, including at least one multiple-baseline design or at least one controlled trial. We divided each set of CAM studies into treatments for chronic or acute/procedural pain and then further subdivided each of these groups by specific condition (e.g., pediatric migraine). We also consider the methodological limitations of the studies reviewed, as well as the some of the major difficulties with conducting treatment outcome research in this area.

2. CAM Approaches for Pediatric Pain

2.1. Acupuncture

In adults, acupuncture is among the most frequently used CAM treatments for chronic medical conditions *(15–17)*, and its effectiveness has been supported for several specific pain problems, such as headaches *(18)* and chronic back pain *(19)*. Reports of serious adverse effects are rare *(20,21)*. Although the exact mechanisms by which acupuncture exerts analgesic effects have not been specified, numerous investigations have demonstrated that the nervous system, neurotransmitters, endogenous substances, and Jingluo (meridians) may respond to needling stimulation and electroacupuncture (EA) *(22)*, in which an acupuncture needle is attached to a low-voltage electricity source.

As reviewed by Ma *(22)*, early studies demonstrated that the analgesic effects of EA are mediated by opioid peptides in the periaqueductal gray; more recent evidence showed that nitric oxide plays an important role in mediating cardiovascular responses to EA stimulation through the gracile nucleus–thalamic pathway. Several substances, including serotonin, catecholamines, inorganic chemicals, and amino acids, such as glutamate and α-aminobutyric acid, are proposed to mediate certain cardiovascular and analgesic effects of acupuncture, although at present their role is poorly understood *(22)*.

There are few published reports on acupuncture for treatment of pain in children. One of the principal reasons for this scarcity of research is the conventional view that children react to needles with fear and distaste *(23)*. Pediatricians will often fail to suggest acupuncture if they suspect such an aversion to needles *(23)*; researchers may believe that inadequate patient enrollment and retention would prevent them from carrying out an adequate trial of acupuncture in children.

Kemper and colleagues *(23)*, however, found that 67% of children referred to an acupuncturist for chronic pain problems (most commonly migraine headaches, endometriosis, and reflex sympathetic dystrophy) and 60% of their parents thought that acupuncture was a positive experience; 70% of the children and 59% of the parents reported definite pain relief from the intervention. These findings support the feasibility and acceptability of acupuncture for pain relief in children. However, most of the patients in this study were adolescents (median age, 16 years), and only those patients who were referred and actually visited the acupuncturist were interviewed. No information was available regarding the percentage of referred patients who refused acupuncture or the reasons for their doing so. Thus, this study may have overestimated the acceptability of treatment. These researchers recommended further prospective investigations, particularly in younger samples.

2.1.1. Chronic Pain

We evaluated the efficacy and acceptability of a combined acupuncture and hypnotherapy intervention package in 33 children 6–18 years old (mean, 13 years) who were referred to a chronic pain clinic; the most common diagnoses in this group were myofascial pain and migraine headaches (46%), abdominal pain (21%), fibromyalgia (11%), and complex regional pain syndrome type 1 of an extremity (11%) *(24)*. The children were offered six weekly sessions of acupuncture, with a 20-minute hypnotherapy session that was conducted while the needles were in place. Only 2 patients refused treatment, and more than 90% completed the 6-week course. No adverse effects were reported, and both parents and children reported significant improvements in children's pain and functioning. This study supports the high acceptability of a combined acupuncture/ hypnotherapy intervention and provides preliminary evidence of its effectiveness for chronic pediatric pain. However, the acceptability and efficacy of acupuncture alone, without the addition of hypnotherapy, remain unclear. Moreover, the study was limited by the absence of a control group.

2.1.2. Pediatric Migraine

Only one randomized, controlled study of acupuncture in children with chronic pain was located in the literature. Pintov and colleagues administered either true acupuncture or a placebo intervention (superficial needling) to 22 patients, aged

7–15 years, complaining of migraine headaches *(25)*. Of the children, 12 were treated with 10 weekly sessions of true acupuncture, with needles inserted subdermally, according to the principles of traditional Chinese medicine. The 10 children in the placebo group had needles of the same size inserted in the stratum corneum once a week for 10 weeks. Children, parents, and nurse raters who administered the pain measures were all blinded to study group assignment. No children received prophylactic medications.

Blood samples were taken from all children to examine treatment effects on plasma panopioid activity and levels of β-endorphin because dysregulation of the endogenous opioid antinociceptive system has been hypothesized as a possible factor in migraine *(26,27)*. The true acupuncture group reported reductions in migraine frequency and severity, and panopioid activity in plasma, and β-endorphin levels also rose significantly. No such changes were observed in the placebo group. These findings, in a rigorously designed study, provide good evidence to support the efficacy of acupuncture in the treatment of pediatric migraine. However, there are several caveats. First, the sample sizes were relatively small. Second, although many pediatric migraine patients receive regular, prophylactic, or as-needed medications, all such patients were excluded from this study. Thus, the study sample may not be representative of pediatric migraine patients. Third, these investigators reported no information on refusal rates, so it is not possible to determine the acceptability of the treatment. Finally, no follow-up data were presented, and it is not known whether or how long after the study the treatment gains persisted.

In summary, acupuncture may be designated as possibly efficacious for pediatric migraine specifically based on evidence from the Pintov et al. study *(25)* and as a promising therapy for chronic pediatric pain in general from existing evidence according to the 1995 Task Force criteria. No published studies to date have examined the use of acupuncture for acute pain in children. More research is required to establish the efficacy and acceptability of acupuncture for a range of pain problems in children.

2.2. Biofeedback

The majority of the studies published since the 1980s on biofeedback (BFB) for pediatric pain have focused on pediatric migraine and a few on tension headache. The most frequently studied BFB modality for migraine is skin temperature or thermal biofeedback (TBF; volitional handwarming), which typically involves monitoring visual or auditory feedback from a thermistor placed on the fingers. Because migraine has been viewed as primarily vascular in nature *(28)*, TBF was thought to be an appropriate intervention because of its ability to have an impact on the vascular system *(29)* via the effects of volitional control of body temperature on vasoconstriction and vasodilation *(30)*.

The modality most often studied for tension headaches is electromyographic biofeedback (EMG-BFB), which again monitors visual or auditory feedback, in this case from electrical impulses generated from the frontalis (forehead) muscle *(31)*. As opposed to migraine, tension headaches have been viewed as arising secondary to sustained muscle contraction *(32)*; therefore, EMG-BFB was thought to be appropriate because of its ability to reduce muscle tension *(33)*. Recent conceptualizations of a continuum model *(34,35)* in which both migraine and tension headaches involve vascular and muscular components *(36)*, however, have modified the application of BFB for head pain in children (discussed in the next Subheading).

2.2.1. Chronic Pain

2.2.1.1. PEDIATRIC MIGRAINE

Hermann and Blanchard *(28)*, maintained that TBF for pediatric migraine may be considered possibly efficacious according to the 1995 Task Force criteria. Their comprehensive review of 15 studies that used TBF alone or in combinations with other modalities found that TBF does not qualify as a well-established treatment in children (as it does in adults) because none of the studies demonstrated superiority over a credible placebo condition or alternative interventions. On the other hand, more than two-thirds of pediatric migraine patients treated in the 15 studies could be considered as achieving successful outcomes based on the widely accepted criterion of a 50% reduction in headache symptoms *(37)*.

A later study by Scharff and colleagues *(38)* compared TBF (handwarming biofeedback [HWB]) to an attention placebo (handcooling biofeedback [HCB]) and a wait-list group. Thirty-six children (mean age, 12.8 years) with pediatric migraine were randomly assigned to one of the three study groups. The HWB group received four 1-hour sessions of HWB as part of a stress management package consisting of 30 minutes of TBF training, progressive muscle relaxation (PMR), imagery training of warm places and vasodilation, and instruction in deep breathing. The HCB group received four 1-hour sessions consisting of 30 minutes of HCB, including handcooling strategies, such as imagery of cold places and peripheral vasoconstriction, and 30 minutes of general discussion with the therapist as a control for the time and attention spent on stress management in the HWB group. All groups self-monitored their headaches to establish baseline symptoms during a 2-week preintervention period. The wait-list group continued to monitor their headaches for 8 weeks prior to starting treatment. Scharff and colleagues found that 53.8% of the HWB group achieved 50% or greater reduction in symptoms at posttreatment, and at 3- and 6-month follow-up compared with only 10% of the HCB group reporting a comparable reduction. The wait-list group showed no significant changes during the monitoring period.

These findings by Scharff et al. *(38)*, demonstrating a clinically significant improvement with TBF, are consistent with existing published evidence of its efficacy in pediatric migraine. However, this study employed TBF as part of an overall treatment package that included several other components; thus, it is not possible to attribute the symptom reduction to the feedback modality alone. Additional work comparing results in a group using TBF alone to a control group receiving a credible attention placebo or an established treatment will be required to meet the 1995 Task Force criteria for an EST. Further, the limited available data on the natural course of pediatric migraine suggest that children may "simply grow out" of this disorder as they get older or respond positively to other nonspecific factors in their environment. Several studies have shown that improvements following TBF persist for up to 1 yr, but as discussed by Hermann and Blanchard *(28)*, the possibility that these may be caused by alternative factors outside the clinical setting cannot be completely ruled out *(39)*.

2.2.1.2. TENSION HEADACHE

Relatively few investigations have been conducted on the effects of BFB on tension headaches in children. Hermann and Blanchard *(28)* attributed this paucity of studies to lower demand for treatment, compared with pediatric migraine, because of relative infrequency of tension headaches or lower degrees of concern in parents and children. In addition, the natural course of tension headaches is likely to be more variable, including longer intervals of symptom remission, which may reduce demand for treatment *(28)*. As mentioned, most of the existing studies on tension headaches have employed EMG-BFB.

In reviewing the three existing studies *(40–42)*, Hermann and Blanchard *(28)* concluded that a "rather lenient" application of the 1995 Task Force criteria would permit the designation of EMG-BFB as a promising intervention for tension headache. All three studies reported high success rates (80–90%). However, none of the three studies directly compared EMG-BFB with a placebo control; two were carried out by the same research group (Kröner-Herwig et al.); cell sizes in all three studies were small; and there was considerable variation in reported outcomes, as discussed by Hermann and Blanchard. Moreover, both the studies by the Kröner-Herwig group included children with tension headaches, as well as those with mixed (both tension and migraine headache symptoms) headaches, but did not examine differences in treatment outcome based on diagnosis. On the other hand, spontaneous remission of tension headaches (e.g., because of stress relief associated with change in school) may be more likely to occur than with migraine *(28)*; therefore, it is notable that in the three existing studies reductions in symptoms were maintained or even improved throughout follow-up periods up to 1 year. Nevertheless, as with pediatric migraine, limited data on the natural course of tension headaches in children indicate that nonspecific factors cannot be ruled out at possible explanations for remission *(28)*.

Two additional studies, one employing a randomized, controlled design, have examined BFB-assisted relaxation as an intervention in pediatric tension headaches. Bussone and colleagues compared EMG-BFB to relaxation alone in 35 patients (aged 11–15 years) randomly assigned to treatment and control groups *(43)*. In the EMG-BFB group, patients received 10 sessions, with the first 4 devoted to PMR and the final 6 sessions using EMG-BFB to assist with relaxation. The control group was simply instructed to remain calm and to become more relaxed during the 10-session program. Although the groups reported equivalent symptom reduction at 1-month posttreatment, the EMG-BFB group experienced significantly greater reductions in symptoms at 6- and 12-month follow-up compared with the control group. However, the EMG-BFB condition was a combined intervention with PMR, and therefore it is not possible to attribute improvements to either of the components. Direct comparison of EMG-BFB alone to a credible placebo is required if this CAM intervention is to achieve EST status as a treatment for tension headaches in children.

As discussed, more recent conceptualizations propose a continuum model *(34,35)* in which the pathophysiology of both migraine and tension headaches involve vascular as well as muscular components *(36)*. Thus, Arndorfer and Allen have lately used a multiple-baseline design to assess TBF in the treatment of tension headaches in five children (aged 8–14 years) *(44)*. The patients participated in four sessions devoted to TBF training and in two follow-up/problem-solving sessions. Results indicated clinically significant reductions in symptoms for all five children. Again, the TBF intervention was part of a treatment package. The children's parents received guidelines for support of independent pain behavior management, and as-needed pain medications were allowed. In sum, TBF may be considered a promising intervention in pediatric tension headaches, but more carefully controlled between-group studies are needed for it to be designated as an EST.

2.2.2. Other Pain Problems

The effects of BFB on other pain problems in children are not well studied, perhaps because it is less clear which modifiable physiological response may be clearly linked to disease-related (e.g., cancer) or other pediatric pain problems (e.g., recurrent abdominal pain) *(28)*. There have been two studies using BFB interventions in treatment packages for conditions other than headache. In one study, eight children with juvenile arthritis who received PMR, EMB-BFB, and TBF while their parents were given pain management training achieved moderate pain relief *(45)*. In the second, significant reductions in pain and in self-treated pain episodes were reported for eight children with sickle cell disease who participated in BFB-assisted relaxation sessions, including EMG-BFB and TBF; however, there was no change in the number of hospital-treated pain crises *(46)*. Treatment response to BFB may well be mediated by psychological factors (e.g., perceived self-efficacy); it would follow that self-control may be as significant as relaxation, or more so, in relieving children's pain. If such mediation can be demonstrated, BFB may receive more attention as an intervention for pain problems other than headache, as pointed out by Hermann and Blanchard *(28)*.

2.3. Creative Arts

Music therapy, art therapy, movement/dance therapy, or any therapeutic interventions involving the creative arts have rarely been evaluated in controlled trials, despite case studies *(47)* and uncontrolled investigations *(48)* describing their benefits for pain management in children. Most of the published studies comparing a creative arts intervention to a control have evaluated live or recorded music as a form of distraction for children undergoing acute procedural pain. Engaging in any task demanding attention, such as listening to music, probably limits a child's capacity to process pain, reduces pain sensitivity *(49)*, and may thereby assist the child to habituate to repeated painful stimuli *(50)*.

There is no evidence, however, that music functions as a better distraction than other stimuli or activities that engage attention, and it has not been established that music has any other pain-relieving or desensitizing effects. Almost any kind of auditory stimulus, including conversation, a cat's purr, or even street noise, will distract a child to some extent; an appropriate placebo is thus essential in evaluating a musical intervention. Yet, as discussed in the next Subheading, few studies have included such a control condition.

2.3.1. Procedural Pain

Four reports of music distraction studies are discussed. Fowler-Kerry and Lander *(51)* evaluated this intervention in a controlled trial of 200 children aged 4.5–6.5 years subjected to injection pain. One group of children listened to music played over headphones before and during injection; a second received a verbal suggestion that the experimenter would help the child during the injection; a third was given music distraction plus suggestion; a placebo control group was given headphones without music, and a second control group received no intervention. Pain was assessed using a 4-point visual analog scale, the psychometric properties of which were not reported. The music distraction group reported less pain on this scale than the suggestion-only group, and there was no incremental effect on pain when suggestion was added to music distraction. The use of a validated scale and the inclusion of an auditory distraction condition (e.g., white noise) would have improved this otherwise strong study design.

In a more recent study *(52)*, investigators played lullabies to one group of children aged 3–6 years receiving immunizations; a control group received no intervention. The lullaby group showed less distress, but there were no differences in reported pain or in physiological response. The total number of subjects was 99, but it was unfortunately not stated whether the groups were randomly assigned, whether the observers rating distress were blinded, or which measures they used. Nonrandom assignment increases the likelihood that chance differences between groups may affect the observed variation in distress; nonblinded assessment may introduce an unknown level of subjective bias into the observer ratings.

In a third study, 20 children aged 0–7 years listened to live music while undergoing intravenous starts, venipunctures, injections, and heel sticks and were compared with a control group of 20 children matched for age and type of procedure who did not receive the intervention *(53)*. The music group showed less behavioral distress than the controls both before and after the procedures; however, both groups exhibited the same level of distress when the needle was actually inserted. As with the previously discussed study, the investigators did not report employing random assignment or blinding of observers rating distress in the children. A further methodological flaw was that the nurses and intravenous therapists were instructed to "maintain their normal modes of consolation or distraction" in the control group; these "normal modes" may have varied across providers and patients.

The fourth study *(54)* is a rare example of music distraction compared to other auditory stimuli. In the study, 121 neonates undergoing unanesthetized circumcision were randomly assigned to one of six groups; one group heard classical music, a second heard recorded intrauterine sounds, a third was given a pacifier only, the fourth group was given music and a pacifier, and the fifth group received intrauterine sounds and a pacifier. The sixth group was the control (no intervention). No significant differences between groups in pain reduction were recorded during the procedure, as indexed by behavioral and physiological measures.

In sum, music therapy may be considered a promising intervention for procedural pain if the 1995 Task Force criteria are loosely applied, but studies using other auditory stimuli as placebos and controlling for the effects of other factors, such as anxiety, are needed if this modality is to be judged an EST. However, there have been no controlled studies on the effectiveness of music therapy in chronic pediatric pain or any well-controlled studies of the other creative arts on any type of childhood pain.

2.4. Herbal Medicine

There are few published studies of herbal medicine as a pediatric therapy, despite the general popularity of herbal remedies *(9)* and the likelihood that many are given to children in the home. The only two existing studies that were randomized, double-blinded controlled trials were conducted by Sarrell and colleagues to evaluate a naturopathic herbal extract (NHE) for ear pain associated with acute otitis media (AOM) *(55,56)*. Although well designed, both studies excluded children younger than 5 years of age despite AOM being the most common complaint in ages 2–3 years. Sarrell et al. excluded these children because younger children are not able to report pain clearly and accurately.

In the earlier study, 103 children (aged 6–18 years) with AOM were randomly assigned to two groups: 61 children received NHE at the clinic on day 1 and then at home on days 2 and 3; 42 received anesthetic ear drops (AE) (*n* = 42) on the same schedule. The NHE group reported less pain on day 1 than the AE group, but both groups showed significant reductions in pain across time. In a larger-scale extension of this work *(56)*, 171 children (aged 5–18 years) were randomly assigned to receive NHE alone, NHE plus oral amoxicillin, AE alone, or AE plus oral amoxicillin. The medications were administered as drops and across 3 days as in the first study. Although all the groups showed significant decreases in pain, patients who received ear drops only reported significantly greater relief on days 2 and 3, compared with those who received the antibiotics. However, Sarrell and coauthors pointed out that much of the variance in pain reduction could be explained by the natural reduction with passage of time, as the experimental variables accounted for only 22% of the recorded variance.

Despite these limitations, it is striking that naturopathic extract was as effective as anesthetic drops in reducing ear pain, and that antibiotics had no additional analgesic effect. Notably, there were no adverse effects reported in either study. The naturopathic extract evaluated by Sarrell and colleagues has been shown to have analgesic, anti-inflammatory, hygroscopic, occlusive, and anti-infective properties *(57)*; other investigators have confirmed that antibiotics have only marginal effects on AOM *(58,59)*. In light of their findings, these researchers *(55,56)* recommended that the naturopathic extract may be considered an appropriate treatment for ear pain associated with AOM. Although the evidence from these two studies is encouraging, replication of these findings in an independent research group are needed for the designation of efficacious according to the 1995 Task Force criteria. Currently, the naturopathic extract should be considered a possibly efficacious treatment for AOM-related ear pain in children. Other herbal remedies should be subjected to similar trials.

2.5. Hypnosis

Studies of hypnosis as a treatment modality for children's pain pervade the literature from the 1980s *(60)*. During hypnotic states, modification or enhancement of perceptions and sensations may occur *(61)*. Hypnosis is often recommended as a particularly appropriate intervention for children, who are generally more susceptible to hypnosis than adults *(62)*, possibly because of their greater readiness to immerse themselves in fantasy *(63)*. Although the exact mechanism of action is not well understood, work with neuroimaging techniques showed that hypnosis is associated with significant increases in occipital regional cerebral blood flow and delta electroencephalographic activity, reflecting the alteration of consciousness associated with decreased arousal and potential facilitation of visual imagery *(64,65)*. The observed frontal increases in regional cerebral blood flow associated with suggestions for altered perception may therefore reflect the verbal mediation of suggestions, working memory, and top-down processes involved in the reinterpretation of perceptual experiences *(65)*. As reviewed by Feldman *(66)*, research suggested that activation of a portion of the prefrontal cortex in response to both hypnotic suggestions for decreased pain and positive emotions may point to a general underlying mechanism.

One of the difficulties in the existing literature concerns the lack of agreement over the correct operational definition of *hypnosis*. A wide variety of terms have been used (e.g., hypnotherapy, guided imagery, imagery) to describe hypnotic procedures, and it is by no means clear that these techniques are strictly comparable. For the purposes of this discussion, the experimental interventions in all the studies reviewed are designated simply as hypnosis regardless of the particular terminology employed in the report; the reader should not infer that all these techniques were identical in practice. Clarifying definitions are used, however, in the section on interventions for recurrent pediatric headache.

2.5.1. Procedural Pain

2.5.1.1. PEDIATRIC ONCOLOGY

Hypnosis for the management of acute procedural pain in children, particularly in pediatric cancer, has been the application most often evaluated in the literature. In a comprehensive review, Wild and Espie *(67)* rated nine studies assessing effects of hypnosis on pain experienced from lumbar punctures (LPs) and bone marrow aspirations (BMAs). Patients themselves described these procedures, which pediatric oncology patients must often undergo repeatedly, as the two most painful and distressing associated with their cancer treatment *(68)*.

Wild and Espie used guidelines published by the Canadian Task Force on the Periodic Health Examination *(69)* to rank the validity of evidence presented in each study on a scale ranging from 1++ (e.g., randomized, controlled trials with very low risk of bias) to 4 (expert opinion). Three studies were rated as 2+ (i.e., well-conducted case–control or cohort studies with a low risk of confounding or bias and a moderate possibility of a causal relationship). The remaining studies fell in the 2– category (i.e., case–control or cohort studies with a high risk of confounding or bias and a significant risk that the relationship is not causal).

Of these nine studies *(67)*, only the three studies rated as 2+ *(70–72)* included a control group. However, the study designs were very different, and the results of the three were inconsistent. Kuttner et al. *(70)* compared hypnotic "imaginative involvement," distraction, and standard medical care in relieving procedural pain and distress during BMAs. Thirty children, divided into younger (3–6 years) and older (7–10 years) groups, were randomly assigned to study conditions. During the first intervention, younger children who had participated in hypnotic imaginative involvement showed greater reduction in distress than either the distraction or control groups at the same age level, but no other significant findings were reported. On the other hand, Smith et al. *(72)*, using a crossover design, found hypnosis to be significantly more effective than distraction in reducing distress, pain, and anxiety during venipuncture, BMA, and LP in "highly hypnotizable" children (aged 3–8 years). By contrast, Liossi and Hatira *(71)* found no significant differences between hypnosis and cognitive behavioral coping skills in relieving pain and distress during BMA in 30 patients (aged 5–15 years). Children receiving both interventions reported less pain and anxiety, and were observed to show less distress, than their cohorts in a nonintervention group, who showed no improvement.

In their review, Wild and Espie *(67)* also followed the Canadian Task Force guidelines in assigning an overall grade (A–D) to the existing body of evidence supporting hypnosis for the relief of procedural pain in pediatric oncology patients. They recommended a grade of D (i.e., evidence from expert opinion or nonanalytic studies, e.g., case reports, or extrapolated evidence from studies rated as 2+). Among the methodological issues they highlighted were the considerable variation in ages of sample subjects, hypnotic techniques employed, and outcome measures used, which made it impossible to compare results across studies in a consistent manner or to reach a determination regarding the efficacy of the various approaches used.

Since Wild and Espie published their review *(67)*, Liossi and colleagues *(73)* reported the results of a controlled trial of clinical hypnosis in 80 pediatric cancer patients (6–16 years old) during regular LPs. The hypnosis procedures followed guidelines published in a treatment manual. Patients were randomly assigned to four groups: direct hypnosis (i.e., direct suggestions for analgesia), indirect hypnosis (i.e., indirect suggestions for analgesia), attention control, and standard medical care. The direct and indirect hypnosis groups reported equal reductions in pain and anxiety and demonstrated an equivalent reduction of behavioral distress relative to the control conditions. However, when the patients were switched from clinic-based treatment to self-treatment using the hypnotic techniques, this apparent therapeutic benefit evaporated. The investigators concluded that hypnosis provides effective analgesia in pediatric oncology patients undergoing LP, but that the therapist's involvement may be an essential factor. As only one hypnosis therapist worked with all subjects, observed treatment effects may not be generalizable.

The use of the treatment manual and the addition of adherence checks by an independent observer made this study methodologically superior to prior hypnosis studies. Taking this study into account, we deviate from Wild and Espie's verdict *(67)* and consider the evidence sufficient to designate hypnosis as a possibly efficacious treatment for procedural pain in pediatric oncology patients.

2.5.1.2. NONCANCER PATIENTS

A handful of studies have examined the effects of hypnosis in child and adult patients with burn injuries. In two study samples comprised mostly of adults, hypnosis reduced pain during dressing change more effectively than an attention control or a no-treatment control *(74,75)*. We found only one published trial that specifically examined hypnosis in pediatric burn victims. In this study *(76)*, Foertsch and colleagues randomly assigned 23 children (aged 3–12 years) to receive a "familiar imagery" intervention (i.e., presentation of imagery related to familiar experiences) ($n = 13$) or to participate in social support control (i.e., casual chat) ($n = 10$) during three dressing changes. Trained raters blinded to group assignment rated the children for behavioral distress. Contrary to expectation, hypnosis showed no superiority to the attention control. The experimental group evidenced no decrease in distress relative to baseline or to the level exhibited by the control group.

Foertsch et al. *(76)* identified several factors that may distinguish burn dressing changes from other medical procedures:

1. All the children studied were inpatients, whereas most studies of procedural pain employ outpatients.
2. The length of the burn dressing change procedure is highly varied compared with other painful procedures, such as injections.
3. The age of the children studied was representative of pediatric burn victims but younger than the average for procedural pain studies in children studied. Thus, lower verbal and cognitive ability in this sample may have contributed to the null findings.

The evidence therefore remains unclear regarding whether hypnosis may be promising as an analgesic intervention for the pain of burn dressing procedures in children.

2.5.2. Postoperative Pain

We identified two published studies of hypnosis or guided imagery for postoperative pain in children *(77,78)*. Lambert *(78)* randomly assigned 52 children (aged 7–19 years) scheduled for surgery to a single session of hypnosis of 30 minutes or less or to a standard care control group. The two groups were matched for age, sex, and diagnosis. The imagery intervention, which took place 1 week prior to surgery, suggested that the children visualize favorable postoperative outcomes. Both groups received the same amount of pain medication. The hypnosis group reported significantly less pain than the controls and was able to leave the hospital earlier after a shorter length of stay, although there was no difference in anxiety level between the groups.

A more recent, well-conducted study by Huth and colleagues *(77)* randomly assigned 73 children (aged 7–12 years) to an imagery treatment group or an attention-control group. The treatment group watched a videotape on the use of imagery and then listened to a 30-minute imagery audiotape roughly 1 week prior to surgery (T1); they listened to the audiotape again 1–4 hours after surgery (T2), and a third time at home 22–27 hours after discharge (T3). The control group spent equal amounts of preoperative time with the investigator and otherwise received standard care. Results indicated less pain and anxiety in the intervention group than the controls at T2 after trait anxiety and postsurgery analgesic intake were taken into account; there were, however, no group differences in pain or anxiety at T3.

The study by Huth et al. *(77)* rates high in methodological quality, including use of randomization, an adequate control group, manipulation checks, and statistical control of analgesic intake and trait anxiety. In addition, administration of the intervention was standardized with the use of videotapes and audiotapes. Children in the intervention group were encouraged to practice at home at least three times prior to surgery, and they reportedly did so (mean, 3.8). However, it is not known whether the extent of home practice was related to clinical outcome. Perhaps the main limitation to this study, as discussed in the report, was the inability to include a sham treatment for the control group that would not function as distraction. The investigators considered the use of a sham tape with white noise or simply instructing the children to wait quietly for the 30-minute hypnosis interval but decided neither was feasible because the children were likely to find other ways of distracting themselves somehow (e.g., watching television). This limitation highlights the inherent difficulties in designing and conducting well-controlled CAM outcome experiments. Nevertheless, Huth and colleagues provided an example of the type of research on CAM interventions that is sorely needed. On the basis of this study, it is possible to recommend a designation of possibly efficacious for hypnosis as an intervention in postoperative pediatric pain.

2.5.3. Chronic Pain: Recurrent Pediatric Headache

Holden and colleagues have reviewed treatments for recurrent headache in children *(79)*, including a category of interventions labeled as "relaxation therapies." This grouping included relaxation training, self-hypnosis, autogenic training, and guided imagery. Thus, even though some of the interventions included self-hypnosis/guided imagery, they are referred to as "relaxation." Typically, the interventions focused on some form of age-appropriate progressive or imagery-guided relaxation with daily practice encouraged. Eleven studies testing the efficacy of relaxation/self-hypnosis/guided imagery for recurrent pediatric headaches were evaluated in the review. Two of the four studies that included an appropriate control group *(80–83)* found independently that relaxation was superior to placebo control *(81,83)*; the other two reported no significant differences in efficacy *(80,82)*. Three uncontrolled studies *(84,85)* and one multiple-baseline study *(86)* also found relaxation relieved headache pain in children more effectively than self-monitoring. Follow-up data from all studies showed that improvements generally persisted across various posttreatment intervals *(79)*.

Holden et al. *(79)* also reviewed two crossover studies that tested relaxation/ self-hypnosis techniques against medications for recurrent pediatric headache *(87,88)*. One randomized, double-blind crossover trial compared home-based relaxation with prophylactic analgesic medication in 48 adolescents complaining of recurrent tension headaches. The subjects reported significant improvement following relaxation and showed no further improvement with the addition of medication. Despite these significant findings, the investigators noted that clinical improvement in headache following relaxation was modest.

The second study *(88)* was a comparison of propranolol, placebo, and self-hypnosis in 28 children (aged 6–12 years) suffering from migraine. Using a double-blind design, patients were randomly assigned into propranolol or placebo groups for a 3-month period and then crossed over for 3 months, after which patients were taught self-hypnosis techniques to use independently for another 3 months. Compared with propranolol, self-hypnosis significantly reduced the frequency of headaches, but no equivalent reduction in headache intensity was observed. However, as Holden et al. *(79)* noted, the findings of this study are weakened by the relative brevity of the drug washout periods in this study.

The conclusion reached by Holden and colleagues *(79)* is that existing studies provide sufficient evidence to rate relaxation/self-hypnosis as a well-established and efficacious treatment for recurrent pediatric headaches. It remains uncertain whether self-hypnosis alone, rather than as part of a relaxation training package, has significant analgesic effects on migraine or tension headaches in children, or whether any of the available evidence may be extrapolated to include other forms of hypnosis.

What is evident is that self-hypnosis may be more effective for certain conditions than for others. In the study of Liossi et al. *(73)*, they reported a loss in treatment gains when pediatric oncology patients undergoing LPs ended clinic-based hypnosis sessions and practiced self-hypnosis instead. Yet, Holden et al.'s review found self-hypnosis to be equally effective as clinic-based approaches for recurrent headache in children *(79)*. Foertsch et al. *(76)* found no beneficial effects for hypnosis in pediatric burn victims during dressing change; Wild and Espie *(67)* concluded that evidence of the efficacy of hypnosis in relieving procedural pain for pediatric oncology patients was relatively poor and inconsistent.

The lack of standards or consensus on hypnotic techniques is a major obstacle to evaluation of the published evidence. If future studies are to produce comparable and generalizable evidence, investigators should use treatment manuals that define replicable hypnotic procedures, as was done by Liossi et al. *(73)*. As discussed, the 1995 Task Force criteria require the use of a treatment manual for any intervention to achieve EST status.

2.6. Massage

Several studies have reported improved outcome following massage therapy for various health-related conditions in adults, including chronic pain *(89)*. Massage therapy involves manipulation of the body by combining tactile and kinesthetic stimulation performed in purposeful sequential application. According to Ireland and Olson, although the precise mechanism of action in massage therapy is not known, increased parasympathetic activity *(90)* and a slowed physiological state appear to underpin the behavioral and physiological processes associated with massage.

The main theories regarding the ability of massage to reduce pain include gate theory, serotonin, and restorative sleep *(91)*. According to gate theory *(92)*, because pressure receptors are longer and more myelinated than pain fibers, pressure signals from massage are transmitted faster, closing the gate to pain signals. The serotonin hypothesis maintains that massage appears to increase levels of serotonin, a neurotransmitter that modulates the pain control system *(93)*. The restorative sleep hypothesis holds that because substance P, a neurotransmitter associated with pain, is released in the absence of deep sleep, the ability of massage to increase restorative sleep leads to reductions in substance P and consequent pain *(94)*.

2.6.1. Chronic Pain

We identified only two published studies that examined the specific impact of massage on pediatric pain *(95,96)*. In the first study *(95)*, 20 children with juvenile rheumatoid arthritis aged 5–14 years had a 15-minute session with their parents every day for a 30-day period. The parents either gave a 15-minute massage, following a standardized procedure, or participated in a 15-minute relaxation session with the children. At posttreatment, both children and parents in the massage group reported less pain than their counterparts in the relaxation group. In addition, an independent physician blinded to group assignment rated both groups on pain and morning stiffness and found the massage group lower on both measures.

The standardized massage procedure and blinded physician assessment are strong points of this study design. However, these are offset by several weaknesses, including the small sample size, failure to randomize (or to describe randomization, if employed), and lack of a control group using a physical contact intervention. Sham massage (light touch) would have controlled more effectively than relaxation for the therapeutic benefits of physical contact, while permitting assessment of the specific massage intervention. Finally, although parent instruction in a standardized technique is feasible and cost-effective, the investigators did not report that they verified parents' adherence to the protocol; some parents may have extended the massage beyond the 15-minute period or deviated from the procedure.

2.6.2. Procedural Pain

The second controlled study of massage was a randomized trial in child burn victims undergoing dressing changes *(96)*. In this study, 24 children (mean age, 2.5 years) were randomly assigned to a massage therapy group or an attention-control group. Before a scheduled dressing change, the first group was massaged for 15 minutes by a trained therapist, who touched only unburned skin and followed a standardized protocol. The children in the control group met with the same therapist for 15 minutes of informal conversation. Independent raters blinded to group assignment observed the children before and during the dressing change. Results indicated that massage patients increased torso movements during the procedure but otherwise showed minimal distress; the control group exhibited multiple behaviors indicative of distress, including increased facial grimaces, crying, torso movements, leg movements, and reaching out during the procedure. These results supported the notion that massage can reduce procedural pain in pediatric burn patients following a brief, single-session intervention.

Further studies with larger sample sizes and across repeated procedures would increase confidence in the findings. Again, as in the previous study *(95)*, comparison with an appropriate control condition involving physical contact would strengthen the results.

In sum, existing studies point to the designation of massage therapy as a promising modality for the relief of pediatric pain. For massage to be designated as an EST, several larger-scale, randomized controlled trials using a sham massage or physical contact control group are required. The development and use of detailed treatment manuals, as well as monitoring and rating of adherence to treatment protocols, are also essential to advance research on this CAM therapy. The work of Field and colleagues *(89,90,93,95)* has shown that standardization of massage procedures is possible but is only the first step.

3. Conclusions and Future Directions

Table 1 presents a summary of the available evidence supporting the efficacy of the CAM modalities reviewed here. Most of the CAM interventions reviewed fall in the promising category, with a few considered possibly efficacious and only one (self-hypnosis/relaxation for recurrent pediatric headaches) considered efficacious for a specific pain problem. Because self-hypnosis was reviewed as part of a package including other interventions (e.g., progressive muscle relaxation), its efficacy as stand-alone therapy remains unclear.

Our review clearly shows that the evidence for the efficacy of CAM interventions for pain in children is highly variable in strength and quality. Only two interventions, BFB and hypnosis, and for a limited set of pain conditions, are supported by a relatively substantial body of work, whereas the remaining modalities considered in this chapter have been evaluated in very few well-designed and controlled investigations. Even if there are several empirical reports of treatment outcomes following CAM interventions, the variations and flaws in methodological rigor of the studies make it impossible to reach definitive conclusions regarding the correct designation according to 1995 Task Force criteria. Moreover, some of the designations in Table 1 were based on the assessments of other reviewers; the application of the 1995 Task Force criteria may vary somewhat across reviewers and with our own conclusions.

In general, researchers have too often taken a haphazard and overly intuitive approach to demonstrating the efficacy of CAM interventions for pediatric pain, and a more systematic approach will be essential if EST status is to be established. As Wild and Espie *(67)* pointed out, many existing studies have leapfrogged through the EST process; rather than first demonstrating that an unproven intervention is superior to no treatment or standard medical care, the investigators have rushed to compare their modality to a well-established treatment (e.g., cognitive behavioral therapy). Large-scale randomized studies, perhaps

Table 1
Summary of Empirical Evidence for Efficacy of CAM Interventions for Pediatric Pain

CAM modality	Definition	Condition	Designation
Acupuncture	Stimulation of anatomical points using needles that may be accompanied by electrical stimulation	Chronic pain (various) Pediatric migraine	Promising Possibly efficacious
Biofeedback			
Thermal biofeedback	Monitoring visual/auditory feedback based on skin temperature (e.g., via thermistor placed on the fingers)	Pediatric migraine Tension headaches	Possibly efficacious[a] Promising
EMG-biofeedback	Monitoring visual/auditory feedback based on muscle tension from the frontalis muscle	Tension headaches	Promising[a]
Music therapy	Use of live or recorded music; live interactive music therapy is delivered by trained therapists using voice, body language, and facial expression to engage recipient	Injection pain	Promising
Herbal therapy	Use of herbs as supplements or tinctures either singly or in mixtures	Ear pain (AOM)	Possibly efficacious
Hypnosis	Induction of hypnotic state using focused attention, deep relaxation, imagery, and suggestion	Procedural pain in pediatric oncology Procedural pain in pediatric burn injuries Postoperative pain Recurrent pediatric headache	Possibly efficacious Unclear Possibly efficacious[b] Efficacious[b]
Massage therapy	Manual manipulation of muscle and connective tissue	Juvenile rheumatoid arthritis Procedural pain in pediatric burn injuries	Promising Promising

[a]Recommendation in ref. 28.
[b]Recommendation in ref. 79 for the category of relaxation/self-hypnosis/guided imagery/autogenic training.
CAM, complementary and alternative medicine; AOM, acute otitis media; Designation, designation according to criteria for empirically supported

drawing from multiple settings to ensure a sufficiently large number of subjects and comparing the CAM modality to "care as usual" or to nonintervention must be the initial step *(67)*. If these investigations provide evidence of pain relief from the treatment of interest exceeding that to be expected from standard care or no treatment, then additional trials are justified to achieve EST status by comparing the CAM therapy with established treatments or to a well-chosen placebo condition. Also, because many CAM interventions have been tested as part of a multicomponent treatment package, further studies to dismantle the packages and test the efficacy of each individual component to isolate the effective, or most effective, therapeutic ingredient should also be conducted.

We offer these additional recommendations for future work. First, standardization of procedures through the use of a treatment manual or its equivalent is required for designation of an EST. Investigators have failed to employ such standardization in many existing studies, making comparison of results across studies extremely problematic. The use of a manual will also allow researchers to monitor therapists and ensure treatment protocol adherence, thus preserving treatment integrity. The failure to standardize techniques and procedures for therapeutic hypnosis, reflected in the profusion of terms employed (e.g., guided imagery, hypnotherapy), appears to be a particularly serious limitation in the literature on this CAM modality. On the other hand, certain CAM therapies (e.g., herbal medicine) do not necessarily require a manual for treatment administration. However, there may be problems of varying potency of preparations with herbal medicines.

Second, increased attention should be paid to the likelihood of methodological confounds if randomized assignment, blinding of participants and raters, appropriate control groups, and other parameters of good trial design are not employed. Lack of careful design increases the possibility that observed benefits may be erroneously attributed to the treatment itself rather than to other, nonspecific effects. Many of these potential confounds are specifically addressed in the 1995 Task Force criteria. CAM researchers should employ random group assignment, ensure that participants and experimenters/raters are unaware of group assignment (i.e., the equivalent of the double-blind pharmacological trial), use valid and reliable outcome measures, enroll sufficient sample sizes to achieve adequate statistical power to detect between-group differences, and devise an appropriate control group (e.g., standard medical care). For particular modalities, such as music therapy, inclusion of a truly comparative placebo group (e.g., other auditory stimuli) to control for nonspecific effects is especially important.

Third, the inadequate understanding of mechanisms of action in CAM interventions must be improved through the systematic testing of existing mechanistic models *(67)*. For example, Hermann and Blanchard *(28)* make the argument that if it can be shown that the observed beneficial effects of BFB on pain are mediated by psychological (e.g., self-efficacy) rather than physiological (e.g., muscle tension) factors, such findings may encourage the application of BFB to other pain problems (e.g., recurrent abdominal pain).

Another important consideration is that the safety of CAM interventions for pediatric pain should be carefully monitored and detailed in published reports. With the exception of trials involving herbs/supplements and other similar substances that employ methodology analogous to that used in conventional drug trials, few studies on CAM appear to monitor safety or adverse side effects. Safety considerations should be specifically discussed in published research on CAM in children, and the number and nature of any adverse effects should be detailed.

Future efficacy studies of CAM should also consider the guidelines in the Consolidated Standards of Reporting Trials (CONSORT) statement, an evidence-based approach to improve the quality of reports of randomized clinical trials (http://www.consort-statement.org/). The CONSORT statement has been adopted by several prominent medical journals, and additional behavioral medicine-specific guidelines have been proposed (97). The five additional CONSORT requirements for reporting on behavioral medicine trials include detailed and specific information on (1) training of treatment providers; (2) supervision of treatment providers; (3) patient and provider treatment allegiance or preference; (4) manner of testing and success of treatment delivery by the provider; and (5) treatment adherence monitoring and reporting (97). Adoption of these additional behavioral medicine guidelines will help ensure the quality of reported findings for trials of CAM interventions in pediatric populations (98).

In sum, it is clear there is a paucity of high-quality empirical investigations supporting definitive conclusions regarding the efficacy of CAM therapies for pediatric pain. However, the studies to date have produced suggestive findings regarding several modalities that clinical researchers may use as guidance in conducting better-designed investigations. There remain a number of CAM interventions for pediatric pain, including movement therapies (yoga), creative arts interventions (art or dance therapy), meditation, aromatherapy, spiritual approaches, homeopathy, and folk remedies, for which no published, controlled studies exist and which were therefore not included in this review. One special group of CAM interventions often used in tertiary pediatric pain clinics but not studied systematically in children includes energy healing, such as Reiki and other therapies that purport to manipulate energy biofields within and around the human body, or bioelectromagnetic-based therapies involving the unconventional use of electromagnetic fields, such as pulsed fields, alternating current, or direct current fields. Many of these CAM treatments have shown encouraging results in case reports and uncontrolled studies; some may have great value; others may be of little more benefit than therapeutic attention and touch. It is our hope that future work may be directed at the systematic testing of all these unproven CAM modalities. The promise of safe and effective therapies that relieve pain in children and may replace or augment conventional medical approaches at low cost is a commendable goal that should be pursued with the highest degree of scientific rigor.

References

1. Eisenberg DM, Kessler RC, Foster C, Norlock FE, Calkins DR, Delbanco TL. Unconventional medicine in the United States: prevalence, costs, and patterns of use. N Engl J Med 1993;328:246–252.
2. Ottolini MC, Hamburger EK, Loprieato JO, et al. Complementary and alternative medicine use among children in the Washington, DC, area. Ambul Pediatr 2001;1: 122–125.
3. Davis MP, Darden PM. Use of complementary and alternative medicine by children in the United States. Arch Pediatr Adolesc Med 2003;157:393–396.
4. Simpson N, Pearce A, Finlay F, Lenton S. The use of complementary medicine in paediatric outpatient clinics. Ambul Child Health 1998;3:351–356.
5. Ente G. Prevalence of complementary and alternative medicine use in US children. Arch Pediatr Adolesc Med 2004;158:292.
6. Rosen LD. Complementary and alternative medicine use in children is underestimated. Arch Pediatr Adolesc Med 2004;158:291.
7. Astin JA. Why patients use alternative medicine: results of a national study. JAMA 1998;279:1548–1553.
8. Bausell RB, Lee W, Berman BM. Demographic and health-related correlates of visits to complementary and alternative medical providers. Med Care 2001;39: 190–196.
9. Eisenberg DM, Davis RB, Ettner SL, et al. Trends in alternative medicine use in the United States, 1990–1997. JAMA 1998;280:1569–1575.
10. Ernst E. Prevalence of complementary/alternative medicine for children: a systematic review. Eur J Pediatr 1999;158:7–11.
11. Grootenhuis MA, Last BF, de Graaf-Nijkerk JH, van der Wel M. Use of alternative treatment in pediatric oncology. Cancer Nurs 1998;21:282–288.
12. Stern RC, Canda ER, Doershuk CF. Use of nonmedical treatment by cystic fibrosis patients. J Adolesc Health 1992;13:612–615.
13. Chambless DL, Hollon SD. Defining empirically supported therapies. J Consult Clin Psychol 1998;66:7–18.
14. Task Force on Promotion and Dissemination of Psychological Procedures. Training in and dissemination of empirically validated psychological treatments: report and recommendations. Clin Psychol 1995;48:3–23.
15. Berman BM, Singh BK, Lao L, Singh BB, Ferentz KS, Hartnoll SM. Physicians' attitudes toward complementary or alternative medicine: a regional survey. J Am Board Fam Pract 1995;8:361–366.

16. Drivdahl CE, Miser WF. The use of alternative health care by a family practice population. J Am Board Fam Pract 1998;11:193–199.

17. Spigelblatt L, Laine-Ammara G, Pless IB, Guyver A. The use of alternative medicine by children. Pediatrics 1994;94:811–814.

18. Melchart D, Linde K, Fischer P, et al. Acupuncture for recurrent headaches: a systematic review of randomized controlled trials. Cephalalgia 1999;19:779–786; discussion 765.

19. Ernst E, White AR. Acupuncture for back pain: a meta-analysis of randomized controlled trials. Arch Intern Med 1998;158:2235–2241.

20. Ernst E, White A. Life-threatening adverse reactions after acupuncture? A systematic review. Pain 1997;71:123–126.

21. MacPherson H. Fatal and adverse events from acupuncture: allegation, evidence, and the implications. J Altern Complement Med 1999;5:47–56.

22. Ma SX. Neurobiology of acupuncture: toward CAM. Evid Based Complement Altern Med 2004;1:41–47.

23. Kemper KJ, Sarah R, Silver-Highfield E, Xiarhos E, Barnes L, Berde C. On pins and needles? Pediatric pain patients' experience with acupuncture. Pediatrics 2000;105:941–947.

24. Zeltzer LK, Tsao JCI, Stelling C, Powers M, Levy S, Waterhouse M. A phase I study on the feasibility of an acupuncture/hypnotherapy intervention for chronic pediatric pain. J Pain Symptom Manage 2002;24:437–446.

25. Pintov S, Lahat E, Alstein M, Vogel Z, Barg J. Acupuncture and the opioid system: implications in management of migraine. Pediatr Neurol 1997;17:129–133.

26. Baldi E, Salmon S, Anselmi B, et al. Intermittent hypoendorphinaemia in migraine attack. Cephalalgia 1982;2:77–81.

27. Leone M, Sacerdote P, D'Amico D, Panerai AE, Bussone G. β-Endorphin concentrations in the peripheral blood mononuclear cells of migraine and tension-type headache patients. Cephalalgia 1992;12:154–157.

28. Hermann C, Blanchard EB. Biofeedback in the treatment of headache and other childhood pain. Appl Psychophysiol Biofeedback 2002;27:143–162.

29. Gascon GG. Chronic and recurrent headaches in children and adolescents. Pediatr Clin North Am 1984;31:1027–1051.

30. Gauthier JG, Ivers H, Carrier S. Nonpharmacological approaches in the management of recurrent headache disorders and their comparison and combination with pharmacotherapy. Clin Psychol Rev 1996;16:543–571.

31. Schwartz MS. Headache: selected issues and considerations in evaluation and treatment. Part B: treatment. In: Schwartz M, ed. Biofeedback: A Practitioner's Guide. New York: Guilford Press; 1995.

32. Silberstein SD. Tension-type and chronic daily headache. Headache Q 1995;6: 97–101.

33. Holroyd KA, Penzien DB. Psychosocial interventions in the management of recurrent headache disorders 1: overview and effectiveness. Behav Med 1994;20:53–63.

34. Nelson CF. The tension headache, migraine headache continuum: a hypothesis. J Manipulative Physiol Ther 1994;1:156–167.

35. Viswanathan V, Bridges SJ, Whitehouse W, Newton RW. Childhood headaches: discrete entities or continuum? Dev Med Child Neurol 1998;40:544–550.
36. Gannon LR, Haynes SN, Cuevas J, Chavez R. Psychophysiological correlates of induced headaches. J Behav Med 1987;10:411–423.
37. Blanchard EB, Schwarz SP. Clinically significant changes in behavioral medicine. Behav Assessment 1988;10:171–188.
38. Scharff L, Marcus DA, Masek BJ. A controlled study of minimal-contact thermal biofeedback treatment in children with migraine. J Pediatr Psychol 2002;27:109–119.
39. Hernandez-Latorre MA, Roig M. Natural history of migraine in childhood. Cephalalgia 2000;20:573–579.
40. Grazzi L, Leone M, Frediani F, Bussone G. A therapeutic alternative for tension headache in children: treatment and 1-yr follow-up results. Biofeedback Self Regul 1990;15:1–6.
41. Kröner-Herwig B, Mohn U, Pothmann R. Comparison of biofeedback and relaxation in the treatment of pediatric headache and the influence of parent involvement on outcome. Appl Psychophysiol Biofeedback 1998;23:143–157.
42. Kröner-Herwig B, Plump U, Pothmann R. Progressive muscle relaxation und EMB-Biofeedback in der therapie von chronischem kopfschmerz bein kindern. Der Schmerz 1992;6:121–127.
43. Bussone G, Grazzi L, D'Amico D, Leone M, Andrasik F. Biofeedback-assisted relaxation training for young adolescents with tension-type headache: a controlled study. Cephalalgia 1998;18:463–467.
44. Arndorfer RE, Allen KD. Extending the efficacy of a thermal biofeedback treatment package to the management of tension-type headaches in children. Headache 2001;41:183–192.
45. Lavigne JV, Ross CK, Berry SL, Hayford JR, Pachman LM. Evaluation of a psychological treatment package for treating pain in juvenile rheumatoid arthritis. Arthritis Care Res 1992;5:101–110.
46. Cozzi L, Tryon WW, Sedlacek K. The effectiveness of biofeedback-assisted relaxation in modifying sickle cell crises. Biofeedback Self Regul 1987;12:51–61.
47. Sundaram R. Art therapy with a hospitalized child. Am J Art Ther 1995;34:2–8.
48. Barrera ME, Rykov MH, Doyle SL. The effects of interactive music therapy on hospitalized children with cancer: a pilot study. Psychooncology 2002;11:379–388.
49. Arntz A, Dreessen L, Merckelbach H. Attention, not anxiety, influences pain. Behav Res Ther 1991;29:41–50.
50. Farthing GW, Venturino M, Brown SW. Suggestion and distraction in the control of pain: test of two hypotheses. J Abnorm Psychol 1984;93:266–276.
51. Fowler-Kerry S, Lander JR. Management of injection pain in children. Pain 1987;30:169–175.
52. Megel ME, Houser CW, Gleaves LS. Children's responses to immunizations: lullabies as a distraction. Issues Compr Pediatr Nurs 1999;21:129–145.
53. Malone AB. The effects of live music on the distress of pediatric patients receiving intravenous starts, venipunctures, injections, and heel sticks. J Music Ther 1996;33:19–33.

54. Marchette L, Main R, Redick E, Bagg A, Leatherland J. Pain reduction interventions during neonatal circumcision. Nurs Res 1991;40:241–244.
55. Sarrell EM, Mandelberg A, Cohen HA. Efficacy of naturopathic extracts in the management of ear pain associated with acute otitis media. Arch Pediatr Adolesc Med 2001;155:796–799.
56. Sarrell EM, Cohen HA, Kahan E. Naturopathic treatment for ear pain in children. Pediatrics 2003;111:e574–e579.
57. Ghelardini C, Galeotti N, Salvatore G, Mazzanti G. Local anaesthetic activity of the essential oil of *Lavandula angustifolia*. Planta Med 1999;65:700–703.
58. Del Mar C, Glasziou P. Acute otitis media in children. Are antibiotics always appropriate? Aust Fam Physician 1998;27:83–86.
59. Thoroe J, Lous J. [Acute otitis media and antibiotics. Evidence-based guidelines for antibiotic therapy?] Ugeskr Laeger 1999;161:5413–5417.
60. Olness K, Gardner G. Hypnosis and Hypnotherapy With Children. Philadelphia: Grune and Stratton; 1988.
61. Kuttner L. Mind-body methods of pain management. Child Adolesc Psychiatr Clin North Am 1997;6:783–796.
62. Morgan A, Hilgard E. Age differences in susceptibility to hypnosis. Int J Clin Exp Hypn 1973;21:78–85.
63. Gardner GG. Hypnosis with children. Int J Clin Exp Hypn 1974;22:20–38.
64. Rainville P, Hofbauer RK, Bushnell MC, Duncan GH, Price DD. Hypnosis modulates activity in brain structures involved in the regulation of consciousness. J Cogn Neurosci 2002;14:887–901.
65. Rainville P, Hofbauer RK, Paus T, Duncan GH, Bushnell MC, Price DD. Cerebral mechanisms of hypnotic induction and suggestion. J Cogn Neurosci 1999;11:110–125.
66. Feldman JB. The neurobiology of pain, affect and hypnosis. Am J Clin Hypn 2004;46:187–200.
67. Wild MR, Espie CA. The efficacy of hypnosis in the reduction of procedural pain and distress in pediatric oncology: a systematic review. J Dev Behav Pediatr 2004;25:207–213.
68. McGrath PJ, Hsu E, Cappelli M, et al. Pain from pediatric cancer: a survey of an outpatient oncology clinic. J Psychosocial Oncol 1990;8:109–124.
69. Canadian Task Force on the Periodic Health Examination. The Periodic Health Examination. November 3, 1979. Can Med Assoc J 1979;121:1193–1254.
70. Kuttner L, Bowman M, Teasdale M. Psychological treatment of distress, pain, and anxiety for young children with cancer. J Dev Behav Pediatr 1988;9:374–381.
71. Liossi C, Hatira P. Clinical hypnosis vs cognitive behavioral training for pain management with pediatric cancer patients undergoing bone marrow aspirations. Int J Clin Exp Hypn 1999;47:104–116.
72. Smith JT, Barabasz A, Barabasz M. Comparison of hypnosis and distraction in severely ill children undergoing painful medical procedures. J Counseling Psychol 1996;43:187–195.
73. Liossi C, Hatira P. Clinical hypnosis in the alleviation of procedure-related pain in pediatric oncology patients. Int J Clin Exp Hypn 2003;51:4–28.

74. Patterson DR, Everett JJ, Burns GL, Marvin JA. Hypnosis for the treatment of burn pain. J Consult Clin Psychol 1992;60:713–717.
75. Patterson DR, Questad KA, de Lateur BJ. Hypnotherapy as an adjunct to narcotic analgesia for the treatment of pain for burn debridement. Am J Clin Hypn 1989;31:156–163.
76. Foertsch CE, O'Hara MW, Stoddard FJ, Kealey GP. Treatment-resistant pain and distress during pediatric burn-dressing changes. J Burn Care Rehabil 1998;19:219–224.
77. Huth MM, Broome ME, Good M. Imagery reduces children's post-operative pain. Pain 2004;110:439–448.
78. Lambert SA. The effects of hypnosis/guided imagery on the postoperative course of children. J Dev Behav Pediatr 1996;17:307–310.
79. Holden EW, Deichmann MM, Levy JD. Empirically supported treatments in pediatric psychology: recurrent pediatric headache. J Pediatr Psychol 1999;24:91–109.
80. Emmen HH, Passchier J. Treatment of headache among children by progressive relaxation. Cephalalgia 1987;7(suppl 6):387–389.
81. Larsson B, Melin L. Chronic headaches in adolescents: treatment in a school setting with relaxation training as compared with information-contact and self-registration. Pain 1986;25:325–336.
82. McGrath PJ, Humphreys P, Goodman JT, et al. Relaxation prophylaxis for childhood migraine: a randomized placebo-controlled trial. Dev Med Child Neurol 1988;30:626–631.
83. McGrath PJ, Humphreys P, Keene D, et al. The efficacy and efficiency of a self-administered treatment for adolescent migraine. Pain 1992;49:321–324.
84. Larsson B, Daleflod B, Hakansson L, Melin L. Therapist-assisted vs self-help relaxation treatment of chronic headaches in adolescents: a school-based intervention. J Child Psychol Psychiatry 1987;28:127–136.
85. Larsson B, Melin L, Lamminen M, Ullstedt F. A school-based treatment of chronic headaches in adolescents. J Pediatr Psychol 1987;12:553–566.
86. Engel JM. Relaxation training: a self-help approach for children with headaches. Am J Occup Ther 1992;46:591–596.
87. Larsson B, Melin L, Doberl A. Recurrent tension headache in adolescents treated with self-help relaxation training and a muscle relaxant drug. Headache 1990;30:665–671.
88. Olness K, MacDonald JT, Uden DL. Comparison of self-hypnosis and propranolol in the treatment of juvenile classic migraine. Pediatrics 1987;79:593–597.
89. Field TM. Massage therapy effects. Am Psychol 1998;53:1270–1281.
90. Ireland M, Olson M. Massage therapy and therapeutic touch in children: state of the science. Altern Ther Health Med 2000;6:54–63.
91. Field TM. Touch therapies. In: Hoffman RR, Sherrick MF, Warm JS, eds. Viewing Psychology as a Whole. Washington, DC: American Psychological Association; 1998:603–624.
92. Melzack R, Wall PD. Pain mechanisms: a new theory. Science 1965;150:971–979.
93. Field TM, Sunshine W, Hernandez-Reif M, et al. Chronic fatigue syndrome: massage therapy effects on depression and somatic symptoms in chronic fatigue syndrome. J Chronic Fatigue Syndr 1997;3:43–51.

94. Sunshine W, Field TM, Schanberg S, et al. Massage therapy and transcutaneous electrical stimulation effects on fibromyalgia. J Clin Rheumatol 1997;2:18–22.
95. Field T, Hernandez-Reif M, Seligman S, et al. Juvenile rheumatoid arthritis: benefits from massage therapy. J Pediatr Psychol 1997;22:607–617.
96. Hernandez-Reif M, Field T, Largie S, et al. Childrens' distress during burn treatment is reduced by massage therapy. J Burn Care Rehabil 2001;22:191–195.
97. Davidson KW, Goldstein M, Kaplan RM, et al. Evidence-based behavioral medicine: what is it and how do we achieve it? Ann Behav Med 2003; 26:161–171.
98. McGrath PJ, Stinson J, Davidson K. Commentary: the Journal of Pediatric Psychology should adopt the CONSORT statement as a way of improving the evidence base in pediatric psychology. J Pediatr Psychol 2003;28:169–171.

7

Technology in Pediatric Pain Management

Patrick J. McGrath, Carolyn Watters, and Erin Moon

Summary

Technology could lead to significant improvements in pediatric pain care. Increasing access and effectiveness of treatment and improving measurement are possible, but this potential has not yet been met. In this chapter, we review the use of videoconferencing, telephone- or Web-enabled systems of treatment, private computer networks, computer kiosks, Internet listservs, personal digital assistants, videos, electronic medical records, and virtual reality in consultation, diagnosis, treatment, and follow-up of pediatric patients with pain patients and education of pediatric pain professionals.

Key Words: Computerized telephony; pediatric pain; technology; telehealth; telemedicine; World Wide Web.

1. Introduction

The major goals of the use of technology in pediatric pain care are to increase access to pain treatment, increase the effectiveness of pain treatment, decrease the unit cost of interventions, and increase the accuracy of measurement, thereby facilitating the evaluation of treatments. Since 1980, much of our world has been transformed by technology. Most of us use the World Wide Web daily to book airline flights, do our banking, buy merchandise, and find information. Many university classes are taught using Web technology. Almost all term papers are written with information obtained from the Web, and professors check these term papers on the Web for plagiarism. Most of our new major appliances and automobiles have embedded computers, and our children spend hours playing video games. Even the production of this book has been transformed by technology. Computers have revolutionized the way we work, the way we learn, and the way we play.

Our health care system uses technology in the form of sophisticated imaging equipment and accounting systems. Word-processing computers are used instead

From: *Bringing Pain Relief to Children: Treatment Approaches*
Edited by: G. A. Finley, P. J. McGrath, and C. T. Chambers © Humana Press Inc., Totowa, NJ

of typewriters, and we develop drugs using sophisticated computer models. However, most of the time, from a technology perspective, health care operates much the same as it operated 50 years ago.

For example, if a child has a medical problem, the child will be taken to his or her family physician by a parent. If the problem cannot be solved in primary care, the physician will dictate a referral to a specialist. The child and family will drive to the appointment and will meet face to face with the specialist team. Unless the child is booked for a magnetic resonance imaging appointment or uses patient-controlled analgesia or biofeedback, technology will not significantly alter care. Although some health centers have switched to an integrated electronic health record (EHR), this is not yet the norm in Canada or the United States.

In this chapter, we review the role of technology in pediatric pain treatment, as well as the way technology can affect pediatric pain patients. We also discuss the barriers that may prevent technology from adoption in this field. Because there is only a small body of literature on technology in pediatric pain, we draw on literature from other areas and speculate about what could be done. This chapter is as much an invitation to move the field forward as a review of the current literature.

2. Prosthetic and Transformative Technology

Conceptually, technology can work as prosthesis by extending the work of a health professional without significantly altering the work that is done. For example, in its simplest sense, use of a computer to type a letter is not much different from using a typewriter. Similarly, looking up a research paper on the computer is not fundamentally different from what researchers used to do in looking up references in volumes of the paper-based version of PubMed or Medline that was called Index Medicus, which began in the 1870s.

Even videoconferencing with a patient in a distant hospital or doctor's office may be best thought of as a prosthesis to overcome distance. A pain team in a specialist center could interview an adolescent with chronic pain using video-conferencing. If the child is in a regional health center and accompanied by an advanced practice nurse or physician, the specialist could even conduct a distance physical examination. The specialist could examine lab results or an X-ray. The advantages of this type of approach are that the adolescent and family do not have to travel to the specialist center. In rural areas of Canada, patients might be several hundred kilometers from specialist care. If the family was in a northern area, it could mean a 3-day trip by air to visit a specialist center. Videoconferencing in this way does not fundamentally change the interaction—there is nothing new about the interview. Although evaluations of videoconferencing in the delivery of pediatric pain management have not been published, the results from other areas (1) suggest that it would work well.

Prosthetic technology can become transformative, changing the nature of the work and the nature of relationships between patients and the health care system. The change from prosthetic to transformative technology is often gradual and unnoticed. So, for example, the ability of a patient to look up information on the Internet is, in some ways, no different from the ability to look at medical texts and journal articles in the local medical library. It becomes transformative of the relationship between patients and health care providers when the patient can readily access all forms of information instantly in the home. About 30% of searches on Medline are performed by the general public *(2)*. When the patient comes into an appointment with pages of Internet printouts and has read the latest Cochrane review of their problem, the balance of knowledge may shift. It is not unusual for patients to have read the most recent scientific articles before their doctor has had a chance to do so. In these circumstances, the balance of power begins to shift.

Similarly, if care can be accessed when convenient for the patient and in a way that the patient chooses, the dependence of patients on health professionals is reduced. When care becomes informed more by evidence that is available to all than by the bias of the health professional, the patient gains more power.

For some interventions, the shift is to self-managed treatment. With self-managed care, the patient is directing and often administering the interventions. The professional may become a consultant or not be involved at all. At the minimalist end, from a technology point of view, self-managed care might involve a book, pamphlet, or manual with carefully worked out sequences of exercises and material for the patient or patient's family. Technologically more sophisticated self-managed care could include use of personalized Web pages.

It is our view that technology can dramatically change the nature of health care and the relationships between patients and health care professionals by giving patients more information about, and control over, their health care.

2.1. Technology Options for Pediatric Pain Care

The major types of technology that could be used in pediatric pain treatment are videoconferencing, telephone- or Web-enabled systems of treatment, private computer networks, computer kiosks, Internet Listservs, personal digital assistants (PDAs), videos, electronic medical records, and virtual reality. Pediatric pain professionals and patients can use these methods for consultation, diagnosis, education, treatment, and follow-up.

2.1.1. Real-Time Contact: Videoconferencing

Videoconferencing uses electronic links to two or more individuals or groups to enable real-time video and audio communication. At its simplest, videoconferencing can be used over telephone or telecommunication lines with camera and audio receivers and transmitters at each end. Web cams and microphones are readily available. At the high end, designated videoconferencing facilities are available at many institutions using fixed facilities with high bandwidth providing very good video and voice transmission, particularly for consultation and diagnostic sessions. Newer low-end, Internet-based videoconferencing solutions using individual camera and voice feeds cost less than $100 per station and offer good performance for informal meetings and feedback sessions between patients and clinicians or coaches.

Videoconferencing provides a social aspect to the distance experience that includes the ability to interpret reactions and nonverbal gestures, which may be especially important when the participants have not previously met *(3)*. The value of the video component, which is the most expensive component, should be considered carefully. For example, in diagnostic or treatment sessions, high-quality video has significant value; for consultative or feedback sessions, the quality of the video is less important. In both cases, however, high-quality audio is necessary for user satisfaction with the interaction.

Videoconferencing has been used successfully for consultations, patient education, regular appointments, and discharge planning for some time *(4)*. For example, our colleagues have been using videoconferencing to provide consultations from Halifax to Amman Jordan (Chapter 8). Videoconferencing has a history of use in distance health care, and studies indicated that patients find videoconferencing generally acceptable and reported their experiences using this technology are satisfactory *(3)*.

Very few examples of pain care delivery by videoconferencing have been reported. The Monash Ageing Research Centre in Melbourne, Australia *(5)*, reported on pain consults to 19 nursing home residents with osteoarthritis and rheumatoid arthritis who ranged from 71 to 95 years. They used telephone-based videoconferencing systems. The residents were very satisfied (53%) or satisfied (40%) with the consultations, and almost all were willing to participate in a videoconference again (93%). They found the consultations useful (94%), and most (71%) preferred the videoconferencing to face-to-face consultation *(5)*.

Especially for regular appointments during the treatment phase, there can be considerable advantages to videoconferencing, in both convenience and completion of treatment. For the patients, there are savings in terms of the costs of transportation and time. The cost for a family to travel from home to a specialty center can be considerable and includes not only transportation, but also meals, parking, and time off work. The cost and inconvenience of travel to the clinical setting may become enough of a barrier that the patient does not complete the treatment. On the other hand, from the health system point of view, the cost of the treatment now includes the cost of the technology and the operating costs, which may not be recoverable from third-party payers. Experiences using videoconferencing in other settings indicated that its use brings real benefits only when the technology is robust and trivially easy to use.

2.2. Telephone Systems

2.2.1. Telephone-Enabled Interventions

The telephone is still by far the most widely used communication technology, and both traditional use and computerized telephony have widespread possibilities for the delivery of pediatric pain care. Most clinical services regularly use the telephone to make appointments and to follow up with patients.

Family Help, a research program that we are currently conducting, is an example of the traditional use of telephones (6). As part of the Family Help program, we are delivering a module on pain that is designed to treat headaches (both migraine and tension-type headaches) and recurrent abdominal pain in adolescents. Family Help employs a user-friendly handbook, videotapes, and a nonprofessional coach who speaks to the adolescent patient weekly on the telephone to encourage participation in the program and to problem solve any difficulties. The coach and the participant work their way through a series of chapters on different topics that include education about the pain problem, the teaching of stress management skills, and other aspects of treatment. The coach reviews with the participant the material that the participant has read in the handbook or has seen on the videotapes. A psychologist supervises the coach. In Family Help, all contact during assessment and treatment is over the telephone.

In an earlier study, we demonstrated that a predominantly telephone-enabled treatment program was effective in significantly reducing migraine headache pain in both adolescents (7) and adults (8). This program used manuals, audiotapes, and a coach. There were several face-to-face interactions throughout treatment, but most of the treatment was delivered by telephone and a manual (9) that was similar to the Family Help handbook. The program was as effective as face-to-face treatment but was much more cost-effective from the point of view of the health system.

2.2.2. Computerized Telephony

The development of sophisticated computerized telephony systems has now expanded the functions available via the telephone. Computer telephony systems can receive and store data from a touchtone phone; understand voice commands; record and classify incoming speech digitally; and synthesize speech from prerecorded files.

Telephony may be used to automate many tasks that are necessary in health care. Biem et al. (10) reviewed randomized trials in nonpsychiatric medicine in which a computerized telephony system was used to contact patients. They found computerized telephony was effective in most trials when used to improve attendance at appointments. Similarly, most trials to prompt infant immunization were effective. The evidence for other medical uses of telephony is sparse and mixed. No trials in pediatric pain were noted.

Computer telephony systems are useful in the completion of simple, straightforward tasks, such as collecting daily diary data and sending reminders to attend appointments, practice skills, or submit data. These tasks have predictable outcomes, and limited variance in vocabulary is expected. The advantage of this use of telephony to the patient or caregiver is that they can enter data at times convenient to them rather than adapting to the timetable of the coach or clinic. Computer telephony systems, such as NUANCE *(11)*, can now be used to respond to more general queries using voice recognition and disambiguation software to identify the question and generate a response from either a database or from a list of set answers to frequently asked questions.

Although most of us have been frustrated at times with computerized telephony systems used in commercial or government applications, there is evidence that patients sometimes form personal relationships with computerized telephone systems with which they have interacted over an extended period of time *(12,13)*. The participants developed strong emotions toward the automated telephone system.

An important factor in developing computerized telephony systems is to build in sensitive algorithms that recognize quickly when the caller is confused, frustrated, or not proceeding and will then switch the call immediately to a coach or other person for assistance.

2.3. Web Systems

2.3.1. Web-Enabled Interventions

Web sites have been developed to provide information to parents about how to manage their children's pain. As these Web sites proliferate and become the main sources of information for parents, it is important that they be evaluated objectively to ensure that they are providing parents with accurate information. Oermann et al. *(14)* used the Health Information and Technology Institute criteria *(15)* to assess the quality of 40 Web sites devoted to the management of pain in children. These authors found that only 9 of the 40 Web sites evaluated met all of the Health Information and Technology Institute criteria. As treatment information becomes more widely available on the Web, health care providers need to become involved in helping parents choose the best quality Web sites to consult.

In addition to Web sites that mainly provide information to parents, some Web-based interventions have been created to instruct children (and their parents) on how to cope with specific pain conditions. Hicks et al. *(16)* demonstrated that a Web-based intervention can effectively treat headache and recurrent abdominal pain. A coach who e-mailed or spoke to the participants on the telephone augmented the material presented on the Web. We have developed and are currently testing a second Web-based intervention for inflammatory bowel disease in adolescents. The program is part of our Family Help program and consists of Web pages that explain the disease and its treatment, as well as Web pages that teach coping skills. Videos model specific skills and attitudes, and a coach contacts the adolescent weekly to help him or her stay on track and problem solve any difficulties the adolescent may have.

Web-based interventions consist of Web pages that inform or instruct the patient (Fig. 1). These can be interactive and personalized or can be quite static. At one end of the spectrum, the content of the Web site may be augmented digital versions of print-based self-administered interventions. At the other end, the content may be developed specifically to take advantage of the Web medium by being personalized, dynamic, highly interactive, and data-capture intensive.

Web-based interventions offer several advantages over print, videoconferencing, or videotape-based versions. First, video clips and animation can be embedded directly into the Web presentation. High-resolution video can be delivered directly by streaming (if bandwidth permits) or offline by CD or DVD supplied to the patient. It is much easier to update and maintain Web-based material than any hard copy solution, especially print or video. Personalized versions can be created dynamically for patients and families and can reflect personal preferences or diagnostic variations. Importantly, the Web, like print, encourages the user to repeat and refer back to earlier instructions or illustrations and to participate when the time is right for them. In addition, the Web offers include e-mail contact, chat rooms, bulletin boards, and the capability to search for additional material.

The automatic archiving of user actions and interactions into server databases from Web-based systems offers the potential for timely interventions, impact studies, and feedback on content. For example, for interventions that include a coach for feedback and encouragement as part of the process, the Web database allows the coach to review the progress of the participant before and during interactions, follow online interaction scripts, and have session notes saved along with data for the patient. From the health care perspective, Web-based interventions offer the ability to monitor progress and track activities, providing opportunities to evaluate the treatment programs.

The cost of setting up a Web-based intervention, once the server architecture is in place, depends on how much new material needs to be created, especially high-cost items, such as video, expensive designs, and graphics. The incremental cost of delivery per unit of service is, however, relatively low, with coaches the

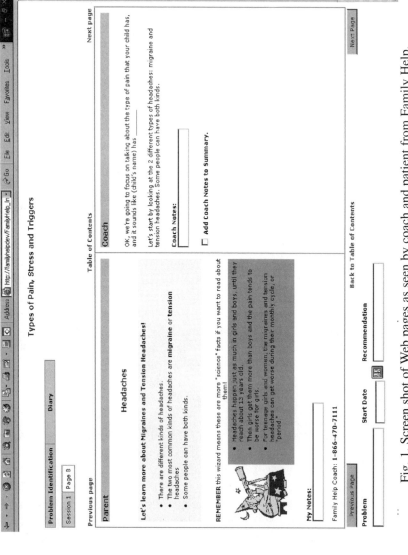

Fig. 1. Screen shot of Web pages as seen by coach and patient from Family Help.

major cost factor. Applications of computer telephony may prove useful in automating many of the low-level coach interactions, such as recording pain levels at certain times during the day or managing appointment times.

Typically, Web-based interventions are generic. That is, each child receives the same intervention. However, personalized interventions are certainly possible with session material that is generated for the user "on the fly" from content and user databases. Web-based systems can present individualized views for users by recording which units have been completed, favorite sections, or personal notes and making this available during subsequent sessions. By incorporating metadata into the content components, such as learning style, age level, willingness to change, or treatment specifics, individualized interactions can be created for patients by pulling appropriate modules from a content database. Further individualization can be accomplished by incorporating specific disorder and treatment data, such as might be kept in an EHR, to modify the content of the intervention on an individual basis. Potentially, the treatment program could learn from previous experience with each patient and with communities of users to personalize the treatment on the basis of past successes.

2.3.2. Private Computer Networks or Intranets

An alternative to the delivery of interventions over the public Web is the use of private computer networks within hospitals or clinical settings for seriously ill or hospitalized children. These private networks may be especially useful with pediatric patients because they allow parents and health care providers to ensure that only age-appropriate information is made available, and that only other children have access to communication venues such as chat rooms.

One such network, Starbright World (SBW) *(17)* was created to allow children to communicate with each other via videoconferencing, instant messaging, chat rooms, bulletin boards, and e-mail as well as to access health care information and play games. Although empirical studies of the effectiveness of SBW are still under way, its creators have found some initial support favoring SBW in terms of lower self-reported pain and anxiety in children who used the network vs children who received standard pediatric care *(18)*.

Although the use of filters and passwords provides some protection for children accessing health information on the Web, private networks guarantee the level of security, privacy, and vetting of content in a way that gives caregivers much more control and assurance.

2.3.3. Computer Kiosks

Computer kiosks are widely used to deliver information in public places. In addition, science museums frequently use computer kiosks to provide entertainment and information. Kiosks are robust and interactive and can be entertaining.

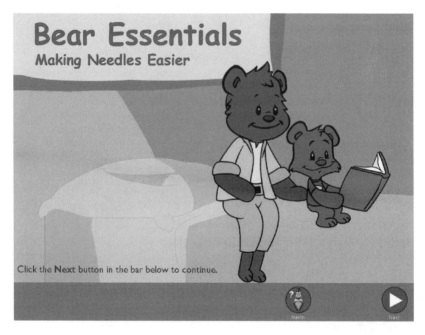

Fig. 2. Screen shot from Bear Essentials kiosk.

They can be available where and when other assistance may not be available. Kiosks are ideally suited to deliver information and training at the time and place that the training is needed. For example, we are currently evaluating an animated kiosk, Bear Essentials, featuring Snickles, an animated bear who learns to manage a needle procedure (Fig. 2). This program is designed to teach parents and children coping skills immediately prior to immunization.

2.3.4. Internet Listserv

Listservs provide an opportunity for communities of users to share information and experiences. Typically, all users (subscribers) can access the "notes" sent to the listserv, and all users can e-mail new questions and observations or responses to previously posted notes. The contents of a listserv may be sequential or threaded—that is, responses listed with the referenced postings.

The Pediatric Pain List on the Internet is an example of a successful use of a listserv for pediatric pain. This listserv was started in June 1993 and has been operating continuously since then. The Pediatric Pain Listserv is open to anyone interested in pediatric pain. Although the majority of the approx 800 subscribers in 40 countries are professionals, parents also subscribe, and many have posted to the listserv. Listservs such as this one offer opportunities for professionals and parents to exchange observations and comments that reflect information that has not yet made its way into common practice (Table 1).

Table 1
Typical Communication From the Pediatric Listserv

A clinical nurse specialist from a children's hospital posted a question:
Could anyone tell me how long the effect of 24% sucrose lasts?
A short time later, a research psychologist responded:
To my knowledge effectiveness duration for 24% sucrose has not been
evaluated. For 12% sucrose, duration is at least 4 minutes, with a peak at 2 minutes
after delivery.
And supplied a reference:
Blass EM, Shah A. Pain-reducing properties of sucrose in human
newborns. Chem Senses 1995;20:1, 29–35.
Elliott Blass
Another nurse joined in:
Elliot is correct, the peak effect is at 2 minutes, and I believe Ron Barr had some
data that showed that it was completely gone by 7 minutes. Many protocols
suggest giving it 2 minutes prior to a painful procedure, right at the beginning
and if the procedure is continuing beyond 2 minutes, repeating the dose. It is
effective that way and seems to be cumulative.
And also supplied a reference:
Johnston CC, et al. Repeated doses of oral sucrose for decreasing pain from
heelstick in preterm neonates. Biol Neonate 1999;75:160–166.

Most of the postings on the Pediatric Pain List are on specific clinical cases
(with identifying information absent) that are posing difficulties in management. There are also discussions of clinical policies and procedures, research,
and job vacancies.

2.3.5. Personal Digital Assistants

PDAs are hand-held, wireless computers typically used to record appointments and keep addresses and other contact information. Many PDAs with
wireless access can also send and receive e-mail, do simple word processing,
play MP3 music files, access the Internet, play video games, and take and display digital pictures.

Palermo et al. *(19)* studied 60 children aged 8–16 (mean, 12.3) years with
headaches or juvenile idiopathic arthritis. They randomly assigned participants
to keep electronic diaries on a PDA or to complete paper diaries to monitor their
pain. Palermo and colleagues found that the children who were using the electronic
diary were more likely to complete the diary on more days (6.6 vs 3.8 days)
than children who were using paper diaries. Children made fewer errors in
electronic diaries than in paper diaries, and boys were more likely to fill in
electronic than paper diaries.

PDAs offer many opportunities in individual health care because they are personal and relatively inexpensive and can be used anytime, anywhere. First, PDAs can be used to personalize and reinforce the process of learning about a health condition. Although a Web site may be more appropriate for the presentation of the content of pain intervention or treatment, using a PDA to augment this material with small tutorials, quizzes, and reminders allows the participant to reinforce the learning experience.

Second, the PDA has been shown to be useful as a diary to monitor pain during the day. PDAs can also prompt and remind a child about treatment or act as a coach for techniques, such as relaxation. PDAs with Internet access offer the opportunity for coaches to monitor both treatment compliance and symptoms during the day for possible direct intervention as needed. So, a child reporting the events that usually precede a headache might be prompted to practice relaxation or to take an analgesic.

A third potential for PDAs in pain treatment is as a distractor. That is, the use of games or simulations built around either the treatment or the disease can act as direct distraction agents. Video-style games can also be designed to reinforce learning about treatments and potentially encourage compliance with treatment. Stinson *(20)* demonstrated the feasibility and usability of PDAs for tracking pain in juvenile arthritis.

2.4. Videos

In the management of pediatric pain, video technology has been implemented in two main ways. First, it has been used for direct instruction and modeling of coping skills for children and their parents; second, it has been used for distracting children undergoing painful procedures.

Jay et al. *(21)* compared the effectiveness of cognitive behavioral therapy (CBT) and general anesthesia in reducing the pain and anxiety experienced by 3- to 12-year-old leukemia patients undergoing bone marrow aspiration (BMA). The CBT intervention in this study included a video in which a child having a BMA narrated the steps of the procedure, as well as thoughts and feelings at key points in the procedure. The child in the video also modeled coping skills, such as deep breathing. The authors found no differences in self-reported pain, fear, pulse rate, or anxiety about the next BMA in children who received general anesthesia vs those who received CBT.

Of course, with many medical procedures, a video-based CBT intervention could never replace general anesthesia. However, these types of interventions do have the potential to reduce the pain and distress experienced by children undergoing procedures, such as BMA, and could be offered as alternatives to general anesthesia in some cases.

Research on nonpharmacological methods of pediatric pain control shows that diverting a child's attention away from painful medical procedures is effective in reducing pain and distress *(22)*. A number of studies have been carried out on the effectiveness of video-based distraction interventions. For example, Cohen et al. *(23)* found that distraction using age-appropriate videos was more effective than EMLA™ (a topical anesthetic) at reducing distress and increasing coping in fourth graders undergoing a hepatitis B vaccination. These researchers also calculated the video-based distraction intervention to be much less expensive in the long run than EMLA.

Currently, we are combining video instruction and video distraction in a study on children receiving venipuncture in the emergency room. Systems such as this ensure that instructions are given uniformly to all children and may reduce the amount of time needed for nursing interventions.

2.5. Electronic Health Record

EHRs are, at their simplest, replications of paper medical records. They can, however, be much more and could transform many aspects of health care and health care decision making. The promise of the EHR is consistent and universally available health information on individual patients. The EHR would ensure that test results are properly filed and accessible to caregivers, thereby eliminating duplication and reducing time delays and the chance of adverse interactions.

There are, however, many problems with the implementation of EHRs. At the caregiver end, many health professionals do not have the time currently needed to enter the data. The myriad current medical records systems do not communicate easily, and repeated transformations of poorly designed EHRs can be more cumbersome and error prone than the traditional paper record. New breeds of EHRs based on standards and meta-tagging are under investigation to remove these barriers.

Once the EHR is established in the health care system, improvements for use at the caregiver level can be made. For example, data input can be reduced or vastly improved using bar codes, radio-frequency identifiers, voice, and simple menus. An EHR-based system could use the health record to prompt behavior for both the caregivers and the patients. Furthermore, an EHR-based system could provide integration of data collection and use across the gamut of pain treatments. For example, content of games and Web pages could be driven by the patient's EHR and behavioral models, and data collected from all interactions could be fed back into the EHR.

The EHR could be used to personalize treatments as well. For example, a simple algorithm could be used to prompt the parent for pain measurement of their child and then use a rule-based system to suggest possible interventions based on the pain level. At the same time, caregivers could be notified that this transaction had occurred, and clinicians could monitor pain levels and treatment success. In this way, electronic medical records could become transformative.

2.6. Virtual Reality

Studies of virtual reality technology build on the video-based distraction interventions discussed in this chapter. Virtual reality technology is comparatively more attention diverting than videos, providing unusually effective distraction for patients experiencing painful procedures (24). Because of the cost of virtual reality systems, there have been few studies on its effectiveness as a pain management tool and none that focused exclusively on pediatric populations. In one small study, Hoffman et al. (25) found that self-reports of pain decreased and range of motion increased for seven burn patients (ranging in age from 9 to 32 years old) undergoing range-of-motion exercises with an occupational therapist.

Low-cost virtual reality systems, such as one developed and evaluated by Das and colleagues (26), make it likely that this technology will soon become widespread in the pediatric health care system. Das and coworkers (26) used a laptop computer, specially developed game software based on the game "Quake" by ID Software, a head-mount display with a tracking system that permitted interaction with the virtual environment by moving the head, and a mouse-activated trigger used to shoo the monsters. A within-subjects randomized design demonstrated that the children had significantly less pain when using the virtual reality device in conjunction with analgesics than when pain was controlled by analgesics alone.

3. Cost Benefits of Changes in Pain Interventions

In our fiscally constrained environment, the cost of any change in delivery of care is critical. When discussing the costs associated with pain interventions, it is important to specify the party absorbing the costs. Costs can be borne by the patient and the patient's family, by the health care provider, by the insurer, by employers, or more broadly, by society. Different aspects of pain intervention may be borne at different times by different parties for different patients. In the same way, the benefits derived from changes in pain interventions may be perceived differently by the different stakeholders: patient, family, community, health provider.

Although no analyses of costs of technology in pediatric pain treatment are available, we can project costs in a simple example of a patient attending an outpatient clinic for initial consultation and five follow-up video consultations for chronic pain treatment.

Consider a system in which all treatment costs are borne by the health system, and all costs of coming to an appointment are borne by the patient. Joey is a hypothetical patient who lives in a small town 200 km from the pain clinic and 20 km from his local hospital. If Joey has seven appointments with the pain team (sometimes seeing the whole team and sometimes specific members of the team), he could be seen face to face twice and by video conferencing at the local hospital or from home five times.

Each time he is seen in the clinic, his mother must take a day off work and drive 400 km. They have two meals in restaurants and must pay for a babysitter for the day they are away. If his appointments are in the winter, the driving will sometimes take longer because of snowstorms. Joey's mother's wage rate is $14/hour, and she is not compensated for time off work. Travel costs $0.32/km, and meals cost $30/day. Babysitting for the two younger siblings is $30/day. Parking is $6 at the tertiary care center.

Costs associated with the telehealth option include an amortized cost of equipment at $40/hour and transmission costs at $25/hour at the hospital or clinic. If a technician is required at the hospital or clinic, costs are $20/hour per technician. If the family is using the system from home, the family requires an initial investment of $100 for the videocam plus access to Internet or telephone service, at $20/hour, amortized cost.

The total out-of-pocket cost to the family is more than $2000 for seven sessions for face-to-face treatment and just over $200 for the telehealth-enabled treatment. The additional cost to the health care system for remote sessions is in the range of $325–$425 for the five sessions. The cost equation would shift if the service provider paid all costs incurred by the health care delivery, if the costs for the telehealth equipment were greater or significantly less, or if the patient lived farther from the pain center. Using telehealth options in the current system results in costs shifting from the family to the health system, with the largest savings the family's travel and time off work *(27)*.

The use of videoconferencing for video sessions in a patient's home is possible and economical using the plain old telephone system or Internet services. Because the speed and resolution are limited, these connections would not be ideal for consultations in which detailed visual or real-time video information is needed. However, routine follow-up appointments may be conducted using this method. Secure Internet services and encryption standards must be met as security and privacy issues are a concern with at-home consultations.

Importantly, videoconferencing can make services available to children who would have only sporadic access or no access to a tertiary care center. If the fair cost of videoconferencing is attainable, the use of videoconferencing may have a significant impact on making services available to those who cannot readily access specialists' care.

Analysis of costs is made more complex because a technological intervention can alter access and utilization of care. For example, if a technological intervention increases access, cost estimates based on access without technology are no longer valid, and new parameters must be estimated. As our example shows, technological change that decreases costs for one payer may increase costs for another. Any understanding of the cost resulting from technological change should include consideration of all payers for all aspects of care.

Introduction of any technology that increases access to pediatric pain care is not likely to reduce overall costs to the health system because at the present time access to that care is so poor. Most children who have acute, chronic, or recurrent pain do not receive treatment; thus, increasing access will actually increase costs. A case may be made that the cost per unit of service, however, can be reduced. On the other hand, overall long-term value to the health care system may be reduced by early intervention, and a case may be made that it is possible to improve access while reducing costs of health services per individual over extended periods of time.

The value argument for the introduction of technology for dealing with pediatric pain is better made not on cost saving *per se* but on increased value, improved care, expanded access to care, and real benefits to individuals, their families, and communities.

4. Conclusion

The promise of technology in treating pediatric pain has been made but not yet delivered. As outlined in this chapter, technology may improve access to care by delivering care at a distance and reducing travel time and costs. Moreover, technology may increase access by increasing privacy and delivering care in a timely way. Automation of some aspects of care may reduce costs. Finally, there may be advantages of technology improving standardization of care.

Technology is not a panacea and is no substitute for good sense in providing service. Technological costs can easily run out of control. Also, any need for expensive technology in the home could disadvantage the poor who cannot afford home computers and other technology. Some will find technology confusing and impersonal.

In summary, careful use of technology could extend the possibilities of appropriate psychosocial care for children's pain. Much work on development and evaluation remains to be done.

References

1. Wakefield BJ, Buresh KA, Flanagan JR, Kienzle MG. Interactive video specialty consultations in long-term care. J Am Geriatr Soc 2004;52:789–793.
2. Smith KA, Sequeira E. Linking at the US National Library of Medicine. Learned Publishing 2001;14:23–28.

3. McLaren P. Telemedicine and telecare: what can it offer mental health services? Adv Psychiatr Treat 2003;9:54–61.
4. AHRQ. Telemedicine for the Medicare Population. AHRQ Evidence Reports. Number 24. 2005. Available at: www.ahrq.gov. Last accessed on Sept. 1, 2005.
5. King C, Workman B. Using videoconferencing technologies to deliver clinical pain management services to nursing home residents. J Telemed Telecare 2004; 10(suppl 1):100–101.
6. Family Help. 2005. Available at: www.bringinghelphome.com. Last accessed on Sept. 1, 2005.
7. McGrath PJ, Humphreys P, Keene D. The efficacy and efficiency of a self-administered treatment for adolescent migraine. Pain 1992;49:321–324.
8. Richardson GM, McGrath PJ. Cognitive-behavioral therapy for migraine headaches: a minimal-therapist-contact approval vs a clinic-based approach. Headache 1989; 29:352–357.
9. McGrath PJ, Cunningham SJ, Lascelles MJ, Humphreys, eds. Help Yourself: a Program for Treating Migraine Headaches. Patient Manual and Tape. Ottawa: University of Ottawa Press; 1990.
10. Biem HJ, Turnell RW, D'Arcy C. Computer telephony: automated calls for medical care. Clin Invest Med 2003;26:259–268.
11. NUANCE. 2005. Available at: www.nuance.com. Last accessed on Sept. 1, 2005.
12. Kaplan B, Farzanfar R, Friedman RH. Ethnographic interviews to elicit patients' reactions to an intelligent interactive telephone health behavior advisor system. Proc AMIA Symp 1999;555–559.
13. Kaplan B, Farzanfar R, Friedman RH. Personal relationships with an intelligent interactive telephone health behavior advisor system: a multimethod study using surveys and ethnographic interviews. Int J Med Inform 2003;71:33–41.
14. Oermann M, Lowery N, Thornley J. Evaluation of Web sites on management of pain in children. Pain Manag Nurs 2003;4:99–105.
15. Health Information Technology Institute. Criteria for assessing the quality of health information on the Internet. 1999. Available at: http://hitiweb.mitretek.org/docs/criteria.html. Last accessed on Sept. 1, 2005.
16. Hicks C, von Baeyer CL, McGrath PJ. Online psychological treatment for pediatric recurrent pain: a randomized evaluation. J Pediatr Psychol 2005, Aug (Epub ahead of print).
17. Holden G, Bearison DJ, Rode DC, Rosenberg G, Fishman M. Evaluating the effects of a virtual environment (STARBRIGHT WORLD) with hospitalized children. Res Social Work Prac 1999;9:365–382.
18. Holden G, Bearison DJ, Rode DC, Fishman Kapiloff M, Rosenberg G, Rosenzweig J. The impact of a computer network on pediatric pain and anxiety: a randomized controlled trial. Soc Work Health Care 2002;36:21–33.
19. Palermo TM, Valenzuela D, Stork PP. A randomized trial of electronic vs paper pain diaries in children: impact on compliance, accuracy, and acceptability. Pain 2004;107:213–219.

20. Stinson J, Petroz G, Tait G, et al. Usability testing of the e-Ouch electronic pain diary for adolescents with arthritis. J Pain 2005;6(suppl 1):abstract 861.

21. Jay S, Elliott CH, Fitzgibbons I, Woody P, Siegel S. A comparative study of cognitive behaviour therapy vs general anesthesia for painful medical procedures in children. Pain 1995;62:3–9.

22. Blount RL, Corbin SM, Sturges JW, Wolfe VV, Prater JM, James LD. The relationship between adults' behavior and child coping and distress during BMA/LP procedures: a sequential analysis. Behav Ther 1989;20:585–601.

23. Cohen LL, Blount RL, Cohen RJ, Schaen ER, Zaff JF. Comparative study of distraction vs topical anesthesia for pediatric pain management during immunizations. Health Psychol 1999;18:591–598.

24. Hoffman H, Doctor J, Patterson DR, Carrougher GJ, Furness TA. Virtual reality as an adjunctive pain control during burn wound care in adolescent patients. Pain 2000;85:305–309.

25. Hoffman H, Patterson DR, Carrougher GJ, Sharar SR. Effectiveness of virtual reality-based pain control with multiple treatments. Clin J Pain 2001;17:229–235.

26. Das DA, Grimmer KA, Sparnon AL, McRae SE, Thomas BH. The efficacy of playing a virtual reality game in modulating pain for children with acute burn injuries: a randomized controlled trial [ISRCTN87413556]. BMC Pediatr 2005;5:1.

27. Stensland J, Speedie SM, Ideker M, House J, Thompson T. The relative cost of outpatient telemedicine services. Telemed J 1999;5:245–256.

8

Developing Pain Services Around the World

G. Allen Finley and Paula A. Forgeron

Summary

This chapter examines the state of pain care for children in developing countries. Various barriers to pain care, such as knowledge deficits, bureaucratic issues, and types of pain, are discussed. Potential strategies for change are explored, including examples from a number of projects initiated in developing countries. Action research is presented as a scientific approach to produce change and build capacity for pediatric pain management in low- and middle-income countries in a contextually sensitive way.

Key Words: Pediatric pain services; developing countries; action research; international development; qualitative research; cancer pain.

1. Introduction

Since the late 1980s, children's pain has become recognized as both an important clinical problem and a focus for developmental and clinical research. This work has resulted in comprehensive pain services for children in some (but not all) hospitals in industrialized countries. However, such pain services are not readily available to children living in the developing world, where there are multiple barriers to care. In this chapter, we explore factors that put children in developing countries at increased risk for pain, as well as those barriers that impede pain prevention and treatment. We draw on the minimal research conducted in this area as well as our personal experiences consulting on delivery of pain care in a number of developing countries.

Developing country is a widely used, but poorly defined, term. The World Bank uses relative, rather than absolute, criteria to define low- and middle-income countries (LMIC) as those countries "in which most people have a lower standard of living with access to fewer goods and services than do most people in high-income countries" (http://youthink.worldbank.org/glossary.php). The World

From: *Bringing Pain Relief to Children: Treatment Approaches*
Edited by: G. A. Finley, P. J. McGrath, and C. T. Chambers © Humana Press Inc., Totowa, NJ

Trade Organization allows countries to define themselves as "developing" or "developed."

According to the United Nations *(1)*, there are 45 "least-developed countries" as defined by a low income (less than $900 per capita gross domestic product), weak human assets (a composite index based on indicators of nutrition, health/child mortality, education, and adult literacy), and economic vulnerability (based on indicators of agricultural instability, instability of exports, economic importance of nontraditional activities, and economic smallness). The United Nations groups other countries as "developed market economies" or "countries in Eastern Europe"; all countries outside these three groups are "developing."

The Canadian International Development Agency ranks countries based on human development index (combining three dimensions of development: longevity–life expectancy at birth, knowledge–adult literacy and mean years of schooling, and income). On that ranking, Canada is 4th and Sierra Leone is 177th (of 177; *see* http://www.acdi-cida.gc.ca/CIDAWEB/webcountry.nsf/VLUDocEn/SierraLeone-Factsataglance). The Canadian International Development Agency also provides information on per capita gross national income and purchasing power parity, which helps define the challenges faced by individual governments.

For the purposes of this chapter, we use the terms *developing countries* and *LMIC* interchangeably to refer to poorer countries with inconsistent health care resources.

As of 1997, the total population in the 125 developing countries with populations of more than 1 million was more than 4.89 billion (http://youthink.worldbank.org/glossary.php). Of the world's population, 80% lives in the developing world, and this is expected to increase to 88% by the end of the 21st century, with the most dramatic increase in the next 50 years (http://www.worldbank.org/depweb/english/beyond/beyondco/beg_03.pdf). In Africa, the population is expected to quadruple, and in Latin America, it is expected to double. The population in Europe may decrease by 18% and is aging *(2)*. Thus, the vast majority of children live in developing countries, yet medical and health research has not addressed their issues *(3)*.

We know that pain is still generally undertreated in the developed world for both adults and children *(4–8)*. There is also mounting evidence that incidents of unmanaged adult pain in LMICs are widespread. For example, Muirden *(9)* noted that pain is frequently not recognized or addressed in Papua New Guinea and quoted Dr. Puka Temu, the Secretary of Health in Papua New Guinea, as saying "most of our patients die and in pain, which is not the way to die at all, given the many currently available treatment modalities for pain control in patients." Similarly, while conducting research in Uganda, Merriman *(10)* found that, despite good home and hospital care for patients receiving palliation, pain was not always treated adequately. Recognizing the lack of consistent pain management for adults living in LMICs, we can identify no evidence to suggest that children's pain management is superior. In fact, McCarthy and colleagues *(11)* found pediatric cancer pain assessment and management to be an "overwhelming" problem in a study they performed in Morocco.

Differences in pain treatment and drug requirements are often ascribed to cultural or racial differences. Although there are undoubtedly some pharmacogenetic factors that influence drug effects *(12)*, there is little evidence that there are differences in pain perception between racial or ethnic groups *(13)*. Within-group variation in pain "tolerance" is undoubtedly greater than between-group variation, and the apparent stoicism exhibited by some groups is probably a learned behavior *(14)*.

Maddocks *(15)* stated that the "ability to cope with pain is a required skill where there is a lack of effective analgesia or no money to afford it." Studies comparing subjects of entirely different cultures indicated that, for example, identical cancer metaphors are used by Nepalese and American students *(16)*, and that reactions of anxiety and distress are similarly manifested by American, Egyptian, and Indian cancer patients *(17,18)*. It is known that anxiety and distress have an impact on one's pain experience; therefore, stereotyping a group as stoic may only increase the disparities in pain care. Navon asserted that there is a risk in cross-cultural research of not only ignoring substantial differences between variables but also exaggerating them *(19)*. The findings from our research project in Jordan substantiated this concern *(20)*.

The implementation of pediatric pain management programs in any country is presumably tied to the state of children's health care in that country. There has been little research on pediatric hospital care or outcomes in developing countries. Worldwide, 11 million children die each year before their fifth birthday from pneumonia, diarrhea, malaria, or measles, often with underlying malnutrition, but more than 99% are in the less developed countries *(21)*. Nolan and colleagues *(21)* carried out an observational study at 21 hospitals in Bangladesh, Dominican Republic, Ethiopia, Indonesia, Philippines, Tanzania, and Uganda and found that inpatient mortality was as high as 15% (excluding neonates). There were 73% of physicians and 91% of nurses and medical assistants who were assessed as knowledge deficient in at least one area of child health care.

Although overall child mortality has decreased worldwide, individual developing countries have not necessarily improved child health outcomes *(22)*. The so-called 10–90 research gap (90% of health research deals with the problems of 10% of the world population) *(4)* is at least as true for pain research as it is for any other field, and evidence for deficits in pediatric pain treatment is starting to accumulate *(7)*. Initiatives by major nongovernmental organizations, such as the World Health Organization's (WHO) Integrated Management of Childhood

Illness program, have focused (appropriately) on life-threatening illnesses but have had no emphasis on pain management.

Given the evidence for undertreatment of pain in rich countries, the undertreatment of adult pain in poor countries, and the deficiencies in child health in the developing world, we come to the unavoidable conclusion that children in developing countries almost certainly receive inadequate pain care. Most children in the world live within the developing countries, and as a result, most of the world's children may not receive even basic pain management following injury, surgery, or disease, and there is not likely to be a pain prevention strategy used before medical procedures or diagnostic tests. Increasing knowledge of pain assessment, pain physiology, and treatment begs the question of why children around the world are not protected from pain.

2. Types of Pain

We assume that children in developing countries suffer the same types of pain as those in the developed world, including surgery, invasive procedures, infections, inflammatory disease, and chronic or recurrent pains. There is no evidence that there is any lower incidence of neuropathic pain, headache, recurrent abdominal pain, pain from surgery or minor injuries, or musculoskeletal pain in developing countries. However, there are some specific disease entities that affect children in those countries disproportionately.

2.1. Specific Disease Risks

2.1.1. HIV/AIDS

HIV is widespread in many developing countries, especially in sub-Saharan Africa, and includes many children among those suffering. Gaughan and colleagues *(23)* found that antiretroviral treatment and consequently immune competence in children in the United States is inversely proportional to the severity of pain reported. Antiretroviral treatment has only recently become available in a few developing countries; consequently, many children suffer from untreated AIDS and presumably from a level of pain that would not be tolerated in North America or Europe *(10)*.

2.1.2. Cancer

Presently, the worldwide cancer prevalence is 10 million, and this number is expected to double in the next 20 years. Approximately 2% of all cancer cases are pediatric, and more than 85% of childhood cases of cancer occur in LMICs, which use less than 5% of the world's resources *(24)*. The percentage of childhood cancer cases occurring in developing countries is expected to increase to 90% in the next 20 years because of the increase in the pediatric population in the developing world. Poverty leads to malnutrition and poor-quality drinking water, which in turn influence the rate of toxin exposure and viral infections, which has an impact on the rate and type of childhood cancers. In addition, there may be a gender difference in cancer treatment. In some societies, male children are more valued, so girls may receive later or less medical care because they are not brought to the oncology center by their families *(24)*.

Curative treatment for cancer is unavailable in many developing countries, or diagnosis comes too late, making palliation essential. Unfortunately, despite the attention on adult palliative care, there is no evidence that this has resulted in improved pain management for the dying child. In fact, there is evidence to suggest that children with cancer in LMICs suffer undertreatment of all types of pain *(6,20)*.

2.1.3. Sickle Cell Disease

Sickle cell is endemic in sub-Saharan Africa and in some areas of North Africa and the Middle East. Gbadoé and colleagues *(25)* studied 165 patients with sickle cell disease in Togo. Most of these were children, and about half were from urban areas. None of the patients used opioids for home management of pain from vaso-occlusive crises, and the use of nonopioid medications and hydration was suboptimal. There was no difference between rural and urban settings. Chakravorty et al. *(26)* compared treatment of sickle cell pain in London, England, and the island of St. Vincent in the Caribbean. As expected, they found much greater use of opioids and other analgesics in the UK population.

2.2. Specific Trauma Risks

It is reasonable to assume that there is greater risk of physical injury to children in developing countries from falls, motor vehicle crashes, and other trauma as there are fewer resources devoted to safety standards and accident prevention *(27,28)*. It is common in many countries to see families of two adults and a child riding on one motorcycle, with only the father wearing a helmet, and bicycle helmets are rarely seen. In south or southeast Asia and the Middle East, seat belts (at least in the rear seat) are rare in our experience, and young children frequently ride on their parents' laps in the front seat.

2.2.1. Burns

High population density, poverty, and illiteracy put people at increased risk for burn injury *(29)*. Burn centers tend to be located in major cities and may have inadequate resources even for the local population. Children suffering burns in rural communities may have to travel long distances to receive care. Although most burns are sustained by women aged 16–35 years of age, children are still at significant risk as they may be playing in unsafe kitchen areas where the working area and flame are at floor level. Pressurized kerosene stoves are common, and they are susceptible to explosions or flame bursts, resulting in burn injuries *(30)*. In addition, fireworks are still popular in many communities during festivals, and children are particularly at risk.

Panjeshahin and colleagues *(31)* found that 51% of admissions to a burn center in southwestern Iran were under 20 years old, and 24% were younger than 10 years. Ahuja and Bhattacharya *(32)* analyzed 11,196 burn admissions to a burn unit in New Delhi over an 8-year period, identifying approx 50% mortality. Of these patients, 17% (1920) were younger than 16 years old, and 16% of those had greater than 50% body surface area burned. Most pediatric burns were scalds from hot water or other liquid. One-third (65) of the electrical burns in the population were to children. The management of burns in this center was discussed, but, interestingly, there was no mention of pain or analgesia.

2.2.2. Land Mines

Approximately 110 million land mines have been distributed since the 1960s in 70 countries *(33)*. It is estimated that 15,000–25,000 people are killed or injured every year; 80% of these are civilian, and many civilian deaths are of children. The small size, color, and novel appearance of mines and bomblets make them attractive to children, who may either pick them up as toys or may collect them as scrap metal to sell. Death or painful mutilation results. The International Committee of the Red Cross (ICRC) collected data from five ICRC hospitals in Afghanistan, Pakistan, Thailand (at the Cambodian border), and Kenya (at the Sudanese border). They did not specify how many children were injured, but 35% of mine-injured patients (who made it to the hospital) were children, women, or men over 50 years of age (i.e., civilians). The ICRC estimated that mine injuries require an average of 32 days hospitalization and four operations per patient *(34)*.

2.2.3. War, Terrorism, and Civil Disturbances

Little is known about the pain consequences of war, terrorism, or civil disturbance in children. We are all familiar with news reports of children injured or killed in terrorist attacks or war, although a Medline search with the criteria {Pain[MESH] AND Child[MESH] AND (War[MESH] OR Terrorism[MESH])} identified only eight publications, most of which were not relevant.

Lacoux and colleagues *(35)* published a report on their research in Sierra Leone with a Médecins sans Frontiéres mission until it was curtailed by deteriorating security conditions. They identified a high incidence of phantom sensations and phantom pain, and 100% incidence of stump pain, in a population of unilateral and bilateral upper limb amputees who had suffered intentional mutilation of healthy limbs by machete, axe, or gunshot. Their sample of 40 subjects included patients as young as 16 years. Even infants as young as 2 months old suffered intentional hand amputation (Lacoux PA, personal communication, 2005).

3. Why Pain Is Not Prevented

On the face of it, it is strange that pain is not recognized and prevented. Most laypersons, parents especially, recognize that children suffer pain when injured, and there seems to be a basic human need to protect children from harm *(36,37)*. Pediatric pain advocates have fought many battles, often with their colleagues, to address children's pain management. In fact, members of the public have usually assumed that pain was treated. For example, Anand and coworkers' *(38)* first studies on providing analgesia for infants having major surgery were attacked in the popular press and by politicians because they assumed that all babies received analgesia, and that they were doing an experiment *not* to treat pain. The American Pain Society presents the coveted Jeffrey Lawson Award each year to a child pain advocate in memory of Jeffrey and in recognition of his mother, Jill Lawson, who took on the cause of pediatric pain after discovering that her newborn son had had major surgery without adequate anesthesia.

So, why is children's pain relief not a priority, and in particular, why have specific approaches to manage pain only developed in relatively few locations in the richer countries? What can be done to change this? Although many of our next comments address pain management and service delivery in LMICs, we believe that similar concerns and principles apply in the developed world, as well.

3.1. Barriers to Care

There are obvious barriers to pain management in developing countries related to knowledge deficits (myths, misconceptions), resource deficits, institutional barriers, social misconceptions, and governmental or regulatory barriers.

3.1.1. Lack of Pain Assessment

There is increasing understanding of the adverse consequences of untreated pain, especially in newborns and young children, but this has not translated into improved pain management practice in many centers. A principal goal in children's pain advocacy has been to teach health professionals to recognize and assess pain. Many renowned scientists have focused on pain measurement research, recognizing that this was the first step toward treatment, but the majority of their studies have taken place in developed countries, usually in tertiary care pediatric hospitals. Although routine assessment protocols are in place in some children's hospitals, there still remains a gap between knowledge and action that is accentuated in developing countries.

3.1.2. Misunderstanding or Misuse of Nonopioid Therapy

We have observed an enthusiasm for nonpharmacological treatment but inadequate implementation, at least partly because of insufficient numbers of appropriately trained health professionals. Nonopioid pharmaceuticals are often used inefficiently, and common drugs like acetaminophen or ibuprofen may be advocated for treatment of fever rather than pain. Unfortunately, we have been unable to identify comprehensive research work in these areas.

3.1.3. Fear of Opioids and Addiction

During the past few decades, there has been a strong lobby against the use of opioids, which has translated into a fear of opioids among the general population and health professionals alike. It is only recently that clinicians have started to recognize the value of opioids used in a carefully titrated fashion for pain. Many physicians in middle-income countries, especially specialists, have done advanced training in Europe or North America, but only those who trained very recently have learned to use opioids appropriately for pain control. Consequently, there is a generational effect—those physicians and nurses who are the educational leaders and role models in many countries trained at a time when opioids were considered dangerous (39). Their use was seen as leading inevitably to addiction, and long-term prescription for anything other than terminal cancer pain was anathema. The opioid mythology was passed on to trainees, and the myths continued. Muirden (9) found that nurses in Papua New Guinea believed that morphine was addictive, and that this information was still in print in a current nursing manual. Livingstone (40) stated that in Uganda, "there are still many fears, prejudices and myths surrounding the use of morphine, especially among older health professionals who were taught that morphine is addictive."

Even when opioids or other analgesics would be acceptable in adults, children are considered especially vulnerable. Children are assumed to be sensitive to opioids or not able to tolerate them safely, probably as a result of experiences with children inappropriately treated with adult doses. Some physicians regard opioids as addictive in a dose-dependent fashion and believe that the way to avoid addiction is to give as little drug as possible. Extrapolation of this belief would suggest that children and adolescents were even more susceptible, although there is no actual evidence to that effect. We believe that teenagers particularly are at risk of "pseudoaddiction" (41), which occurs when inadequate opioid treatment for pain triggers a demand from the patient for more opioids, which is interpreted by health professionals as drug-seeking behavior (which it is) and synonymous with addiction (which it is not). This reinforces physicians' practice of giving as little medication as possible.

Even when physicians wish to use opioids or other analgesics, they may be unavailable or a prescription may be impeded by overwhelming bureaucratic barriers *(42,43)*. One of us (G. A. F) witnessed opioid rationing in Thailand, extreme restrictions on duration of prescriptions in Jordan (3 days), and government prohibition of morphine importation in El Salvador in the late 1990s. Even if drugs are available, they may be prohibitively expensive *(9)*. Nolan et al. *(21)* found that 19 of the 21 hospitals in their study required parents of patients to pay for drugs and intravenous fluids *before* they were administered, even in emergencies.

De Simone *(44)* reported that, in a palliative care program in Argentina, people with advanced cancer are able to receive chemotherapy (including second-line agents) free of charge, but they must often pay unaffordable prices for opioids. Opioids may not even be available in the dosage forms required. Immediate-release morphine tablets are often difficult to acquire, and oral suspensions suitable for children are even rarer. The importance of opioid availability cannot be overstated. Anne Merriman was successful in developing Hospice Uganda, at least partly because of her insistence that the government import inexpensive powdered morphine *(45)*.

4. Approaches Attempted

The need for pain management in LMICs is starting to be recognized. However, the efforts to implement pain management programs described in the literature have generally been linked to palliative care initiatives for dying cancer patients and, more recently, people dying from AIDS. There are few articles that addressed cancer pain management for nonterminal patients in the developing world; there is little literature on general or chronic pain management and even less on approaches to children's pain management. Many of the articles reviewed describe similar challenges, including government policy, lack of financial and human resources, cultural differences, and knowledge gaps, especially an overriding fear of opioids. Therefore, the question remains, what is the best way to improve pain management in LMICs?

Several authors have described their experiences attempting to improve the management of pain in developing countries. Most have not used a rigorous research design, and their projects have been palliative care initiatives for adults with pain as a major focus. Nevertheless, we felt it was important to describe some of these experiences as they offer insights into the challenges faced in delivering pain management in LMICs. The initiatives have achieved varying degrees of success. Some activists have tried lobbying for change to national laws restricting access to opioids, whereas others have attempted small-scale demonstration projects. Again, the importance of opioid availability is highlighted in this quotation from Ghooi and Ghooi *(39)*: "A principle of pharmacokinetics teaches us that unless the drug reaches the site of action, it cannot be expected to exert its dynamic effect. With morphine the situation is that when the drug does not reach the patient, what hope is there of pain relief?" Although these authors were describing the restrictive legal situation in India, the same could be said for many countries where unfounded fears of opioid addiction and diversion prevent patients from receiving much-needed opioids.

4.1. Experience in India

Although it makes sense that laws should be put in place to make opioids available, changing the law does not necessarily result in improved access for patients. More problematic is the disconnect among law, knowledge, and practice. For example, Ghooi and Ghooi *(43)* petitioned the Delhi High Court in 1998 on behalf of cancer patients in India and were successful in having the High Court direct state governments to amend their restrictive opioid laws. However, by 2004, only 8 of the 28 states in India had actually amended their rules *(46)*. There appears to be no repercussions for those state governments that decided not to change. In theory, patients who were prevented access to opioids could bring their case to court, but in practice, this avenue was not pursued *(43)*. Cancer patients at the end of life and the families caring for them have few resources of time or money to fight such battles.

Changes in laws must be coupled with changes in attitudes. Rajagopal and Venkateswaran *(47)* found that, despite the change in opioid regulations in 8 of the 28 states, actual implementation of the change has only occurred in the state of Kerala. They also noted that, although palliative care has been included as part of the National Cancer Control Program, there are no specific pain services, no chronic pain services in the Indian health care system, and no major impact on procurement of opioids other than in Kerala. The WHO advocates for three essential components to achieve improvements in cancer pain management: government policy to recognize importance of pain control, opioid availability, and professional education. However, it seems that the integration of these components has not yet been achieved throughout India. What sort of palliative care can be delivered when there are such obstacles to pain management?

Presently, in the state of Kerala, a group of physicians and social activists interested in palliative care have developed a nongovernmental agency called the Pain and Palliative Care Society and are attempting to address issues concerning dying patients *(46)*. It is unclear if this group is the reason why there has been advancement in access to opioids in Kerala, yet barriers remain even in this state. Rajagopal and Venkateswaran *(47)* identified poverty as a great barrier to medical treatment in India because the country does not have state-sponsored social security or effective medical insurance programs.

Although there is some success in the integration of care for dying patients in Kerala, it is unclear how many patients are receiving adequate pain relief as financial restraints and government control remain barriers. If these barriers remain in what some have termed the "enlightened" state, the situation remains grave for suffering patients in the other 27 states. More troubling is that there is no mention of children in any of the articles reviewed. As children have little or no voice, one can only wonder about their access to pain management; even the well-developed palliative care program in Kerala does not yet have a pediatric specialty component (Rajagopal MR, personal communication, 2005).

4.2. Experience in Uganda

Other authors have described their experiences in bringing about a change in pain management by working on smaller initiatives. Hospice Africa-Uganda stands out as a success story in its ability to treat pain in patients dying from cancer and HIV *(40)*. Anne Merriman, a physician with many years of experience in the developing world, and Mbenaka Fazal, a palliative care nurse specialist, set up the hospice as a nongovernmental organization in 1993. Pain control is the cornerstone of Hospice Uganda's program. Merriman has expressed concern over organizations that claim to be providing palliative care yet do not control pain *(45)* and therefore insisted that the Ugandan government ensure the importation of powered morphine for the small project prior to starting. Over time, the government has become very supportive of the Hospice Uganda initiative, which is now countrywide, and since 2002, the government has provided morphine free of charge for terminally ill patients *(45)*.

Hospice Africa was established as a UK charity that permitted the channeling of funds to Hospice Africa-Uganda. It must be acknowledged that one of the possible reasons for the hospice's success is that Uganda has been politically stable in recent years, which ensured that outside sources of funding could be obtained from the parent charity beyond the initial 3 months *(40)*. The hospice has also been successful in securing various international charitable denotations, particularly for AIDS care; however, long-term funding remains a challenge.

Part of Hospice Uganda's success relates to a model of care that suits the context of the country. According to Livingstone, three studies by Dr. E. Kikule revealed that Ugandans preferred to die at home, and a home-based model took into consideration the financial constraints of the country's health care system *(40)*. Hence, Hospice Uganda delivers care using a home-based model and depends on local volunteers, who are trained by the hospice staff in a 3-day course, to provide much of the basic hands-on care. The fact that 4000 individuals have been cared for within the first 10 years of Hospice Uganda's existence speaks to the success of their model and the real need for palliative care and pain management. Presently, there are approx 400 active patients in the hospice's caseload.

The benefits of starting small were many. The founders were able to demonstrate to the public and the government that the myths surrounding opioids were unfounded; the police escorts for morphine shipments from the airport to the clinic, which were initially insisted on, are no longer necessary. As word spread about the care patients received, health professionals, volunteers, and patients wanted to be involved. As of 2003, Hospice Uganda had trained approx 450 non-health care professionals and 937 health professionals through their courses, adding to its pool of committed workers. They received 1019 referrals between April 2001 and April 2002 (40).

The architects of this project found networking with international leaders to be essential. This is not surprising as others have found support from outside experts to be helpful in validation of local experts (15). Hospice Uganda has been successful in connecting with other organizations that provide palliative care and education, such as the WHO and the Aids Support Organization.

The activities of Hospice Uganda have continued to grow; now, in addition to providing direct patient care, the hospice provides training for their counterparts from other African nations in palliative care and pain management. The once-informal teachings on pain management and palliative care have grown into formal university credit courses. Palliative care is now part of the medical and nursing core curriculum at the two university hospitals in Uganda (40). In addition, on average, 5 1-week health professional programs are given each year. The five non-health professional programs vary in length depending on the target group.

Hospice Uganda continues to deal with challenges. For example, although pain control is the cornerstone of its palliative care approach, only physicians are authorized to order morphine. This presents a problem for the hospice as there are many more patients requiring morphine than there are physicians who can order morphine. This is especially true for rural patients. The average physician-to-patient ratio can range from 1:18,700 to 1:50,000, (45), which translates into 1 physician for every 200 patients in need of pain control (10). To meet this challenge, the government has modified the law to allow nurse specialists to prescribe morphine, and as of 2003, the 9-month specialist prescriber course funded by the government had been completed by 17 nurses. Despite the success of Hospice Uganda, there is no mention of care related to children or initiatives related to nonterminal disease pain management.

4.3. Experience in Argentina

In addition to the numerous challenges and barriers already identified, De Simone (44) asserted that fragmentation of the health care system has an impact on clinicians' ability to provide pain control and palliative care in Argentina. There are three sectors that make up the Argentinean health care system: the Public Health Services, private health plans, and the Medical Health System. However, these three sectors act in isolation, and there are no mechanisms linking one to another.

The Public Health Service is the only one that provides free services, and complex treatments are given priority over simple primary health care initiatives. It appears that individuals with certain forms of advanced incurable cancer are able to receive second-line chemotherapy agents free of charge from either the public system or their insurance but must pay for "strong" opioids *(44)*. In most situations, the costs of these strong opioids are prohibitive; for example, according to Wenk *(48)*, the cost of morphine hydrochloride doubled between 1991 and 1992. Complicating the matter, many hospitals in the public system do not have oral morphine, and prohibitive government laws add to the burden of securing pain management. However, professionals dedicated to the care of dying patients have banded together to form the Argentinean Association of Palliative Care (AACP), a movement dedicated to improve pain control and palliative care.

As in most of the situations in LMICs described thus far, progress occurs in stages. The same is true of the palliative care movement in Argentina. During the early stages, professionals were trained abroad, established supportive links with international experts, and founded the AACP. This resulted in the establishment of regular AACP conferences and the sharing of solutions among individuals and groups who care about cancer pain relief.

The latest stage has been the development of bottom-up approaches. De Simone *(44)* stated "numerous small, effective programs made more impact on the status of palliative care throughout the country than large-scale government-run programs that lacked the resources and commitment to adequately implement good care." Nevertheless, the fragmented health care system continues to be a bureaucratic challenge, as does morphine procurement. Pharmaceutical companies do not provide a range of opioids and dosage forms at a reasonable cost.

Again, children are not the focus of care; most of the palliative care teams only provide care to adults *(44)*. Pediatric palliative care is starting to be addressed, and there are now pediatric palliative care teams in a few major cities, but there is no mention of pain control in the published descriptions. Given that children receive fewer opioids than adults for comparable conditions *(4,5)*, there is no reason to believe that children in Argentina are receiving superior pain management to that of adult palliative care patients.

As stated, the literature describing the state of children's pain management in LMICS is minimal. We cannot assume that palliative care necessarily means pain management in some of the LMICs as some authors have noted this to be lacking (45,47). Nevertheless, there are a couple of initiatives aimed at improving the plight of children suffering from cancer pain.

4.4. Experience in Morocco

McCarthy et al. (11) conducted a qualitative study with health care professionals from two pediatric centers in Morocco (Casablanca and Rabat). The goals of their research were to improve knowledge, collect data on children's cancer pain management practice and policy, and establish a research partnership. Data were collected in focus groups with 11 physicians (oncologists and residents), 14 nurses, and the 3 North American and 2 Moroccan researchers. Four themes emerged from their analysis. They found that pain is an "overwhelming situation" for these health care professionals. The physicians and nurses are quoted as saying the "family is always asking … [for] some relief."

There was evidence to support their second theme indicating a "lack of training and resources." The physicians and nurses stated, "If there are no signs of pain we do not look into it;" pain was rarely assessed, and surprisingly, physicians voiced a belief that nurses had no role in pain management. Lack of pain assessment has been found to be an issue in other developing countries as well. Al-Hassan et al. (49) found that Jordanian nurses did not assess postoperative pain and did not intervene when the patient verbalized the existence of pain.

The researchers' third theme was "cultural influences and beliefs about pain management in Morocco," which did not identify a consistent religious or ethnic cultural barrier to pain management. The researchers did find that common but inappropriate opioid myths and practices, including fear of addiction and restriction of opioids to terminal patients, were prevalent among the focus group participants. Inaccurate information about the use of opioids is not specific to Moroccan health professionals or to the Moroccan public and has been identified as a barrier to pain management in many other developed and developing countries irrespective of culture.

The last theme that emerged was the need for a comprehensive approach to pain management. The focus group participants voiced a need for simple policies for pain assessment and management that would take into consideration the available resources. It was clear that involvement of nurses and parents was essential. Administrative support would be required to eliminate institutional barriers. At one of the hospitals, the pharmacy was not opened at night; therefore, analgesics were only available during day shifts. In the other, oncologists had to obtain a special opioid prescription pad that was locked in their supervisor's desk; if the supervisor was unavailable, then opioids were also unavailable. Despite the insight this study offers, there were no suggested strategies for making changes in this setting other than the development of basic policies.

However, the authors did indicate that the research stimulated useful discussion regarding a pain management program for children with cancer.

4.5. Experience in Jordan

In collaboration with a Jordanian colleague, we described the process of implementation of a sustainable pediatric pain program at the King Hussein Cancer Center in Amman, Jordan *(20,50)*. This project originated as an invitation to one of the researchers (G. A. F.) to go to Amman for 3 months and set up a pediatric cancer pain management service. It was noted from the outset that a 3-month stay by a foreign "expert" might not be the best way to bring about real change and implement a sustainable program, so an alternate approach was devised.

It is clear from the examples of palliative care and pain management initiatives that collaboration with the community and authorities is essential. The literature on international health development projects identified building capacity as vital for sustainability of a project *(51)*, and this requires an approach that is inclusive of the local community and engages the practitioners in a meaningful way, not just as the audience for didactic lectures.

But what is capacity building? Morgan *(52)* defined *capacity* as "the abilities, behaviors, relationships, and values that enable individuals, groups and organizations at any level of society to carry out functions or tasks and to achieve their development objectives over time." This can be a challenge as it implies that capacity building is an ongoing activity. For a pediatric pain program to be sustainable, there would have to be local champions to act as role models, experts, and mentors to help improve knowledge, change attitudes, and maintain changes in behavior. Keeping these concepts in mind, we used an action research design to implement the pediatric cancer pain management program in Amman.

Action research is an applied research approach and is described as a process of discovery with the goal of capacity building and implementation of change *(53)*. As its name implies, action research is research that leads to change during, and because of, the process of conducting the research. By using repeated cycles of critically reflecting and reviewing, planning, implementing, analyzing and discussing outcomes data with system members, reaching conclusions, and defining new sets of action plans, change can be initiated *(54)*.

An action research approach has been used and found to be successful in other developing world initiatives *(55–57)*. It is an interactive way of formally engaging local individuals in the research process. The goal is to discover problems and solutions for issues that are important for the local community and through this process build capacity within the community so that when the research period is over the project is sustainable. One benefit is that it reflects the importance of addressing matters of genuine concern and relevance to the practitioners involved, therefore helping to facilitate practice change. In our project, some of the physicians and nurses identified the need for a pediatric cancer pain management program, and they were strongly supported by the director general of the hospital.

We designed three research studies so that information from the first two studies helped inform the process for the third. The first study determined the pain prevalence in children receiving care at the King Hussein Cancer Centre. These data were helpful in not only identifying the magnitude of the problem in their own context, but also assisting in securing further financial and leadership support from hospital administrators. Thirty-five children, representing inpatients and clinic patients over a 24-hour period, were included in the pain prevalence study. The interviews with the children revealed that 47% of children had pain at the time of interview; 11% had "a lot" of pain, and chart audits showed that only 22% received analgesics *(20)*.

The second study was qualitative and captured parents' beliefs and attitudes about pain management through individual interviews *(20)*. The data from this study helped to counter some of the myths that health professionals held regarding parental barriers to pain management. There is little published literature about Arab parents' attitudes and beliefs from a cultural or religious perspective, and the articles we found were not research-based. The expected beliefs that parents would expect their children not to express but to tolerate pain *(49)* or that parents might not want morphine used for fears of addiction were not found to be true for the 22 parents interviewed. In fact, the opposite was found; most parents believed that their child had a responsibility to express their pain so others would know about it, and parents wanted analgesics to be used. Parents never mentioned any concerns about addiction *(20)*. In addition, parents expected their child's pain to be managed pharmacologically; one stated, "psychology is not enough."

The third study took an action research approach; 4 visits occurred over 21 months. Videoconferencing provides interim support for the local participants. A "key participant" group of physicians, nurses, and a pharmacist was identified, and general staff interviews with physicians and nurses were conducted during the second and third visits to determine the present state of pain management, staffs' beliefs about children's pain management, and the challenges they saw in changing practice.

The key participant group determined the model of pain management to be used and decided how best to change the attitudes and knowledge of the health professionals because it was clear that many myths regarding children's pain management existed. A pediatric cancer pain management team was the model chosen for implementation; the members included an oncologist, a pediatric surgeon, and a pediatric nurse.

Policy development and implementation were identified as essential first steps before general education of the staff. Interviews revealed that the staff wanted to know what they had to do before knowing the background reasons why *(50)*. Several fundamental areas of pain management were addressed first, including regular assessment and basic medication administration. Policies were based on the resources available at the hospital *(11,15)*. Maddocks *(15)* advocated that

> It is the demonstration of what can be done locally, and how best to establish it which carries most weight. Do not preach to some hoped-for ideal. Recognize existing local gaps and difficulties and work within them while exploring ways through them. There is little value in teaching the use of opioids that cannot be obtained; explore what can be done with what is available now. (p. 218)

We considered this a guiding principle of how to approach sustainable change. Presently, the pediatric cancer pain management service at the King Hussein Cancer Centre is providing expert care to children and has been receiving increasing numbers of consults. Protocols and policies require staff to complete regular pain assessments, and treatments are based on assessments. The nurse clinician is an essential member of the project as she is a constant presence on the nursing unit and is a valuable resource to both physicians and nurses. The physicians on the pain service not only provide direct medical care for specific children, but also provide education and role-modeling.

5. Where Next?

The question remains: how is it best to bring pain management to children in the developing world? Many of the projects discussed in this chapter are based on adult palliative care initiatives for cancer, and although these experiences shed light on some of the difficulties encountered and strategies attempted, they do not offer a clear implementation plan for similar projects. There is little data about pediatric palliative care and no research on pediatric pain management projects outside terminal illness in LMICs. Even our research only addressed pain care for children with cancer.

Our experience has made us aware that there is a need for advocacy on the international stage. Although there is a real need for an improvement in children's cancer pain management and pain management at the end of life, we have concerns about the concentration in this area. There is no evidence that material designed by international experts (such as the WHO's *Cancer Pain Relief and Palliative Care in Children [58]*) has the spillover effect to non-cancer pain that many of us would like to see. The association of cancer with pain seems to keep pain management strategies in a box.

Although we applaud efforts aimed at decreasing children's cancer pain, the same strategies are rarely used for other types of pain. For example, many in Western hospitals use the WHO cancer pain analgesic ladder as a guide to managing other types of pain, but we have found no evidence that this occurs in most LMICs. In fact, the word *cancer* in the title of the manual seems to make the content nontransferable to other pain situations. On our first visit to King Hussein Cancer Centre, there was little transfer of knowledge or techniques from pediatric cancer pain to surgical pain management. There was a voiced belief during the staff interviews that treating cancer pain is a legitimate use of analgesics, especially opioids, but treating other pain is not. Even in this situation, intravenous morphine infusions were only for "dying patients." Investigating and treating the source of symptoms, such as pain, take precedence over relieving suffering *(59)*.

So, where do we go from here? One strategy would be for international organizations to disseminate explicit position statements on children's pain management so that clinicians in LMICs would have support for their own initiatives. It is important to remember that policies and standards of practice in Western hospitals may not be transferable to LMICs. Maddocks *(15)* noted that, although there are well-developed criteria and curricula for palliative care education in the Western world, "Neither content nor teaching method for those developments can be assumed to be relevant to poorer countries with quite different health care needs, cultures, and health care systems." The same principles undoubtedly apply to children's pain management. Although it may be exciting for "rich country" experts to visit and lecture in developing countries, it is necessary to deliver practical information, not just report on what we do in our settings.

It is clear that more research is needed: "Processes that lead to change in high income settings may not easily be replicated in health facilities in low income countries" *(60)*. Although our action research project has had some success, this approach may be a relatively long and expensive venture for some LMICs. Yet, innovative action research projects, as well as local projects involving audits and case studies, contribute important information about the factors that influence change *(60)*. Neufeld reminded us that "global health research should effect change in LMICs" where resources are scarce *(61)*. This position was echoed by Garner and colleagues, who believe that resource shortages should not deter attempts to provide evidence-based care, but that careful consideration is required to bring about small and incremental changes *(60)*.

On October 17, 2005, the International Association for the Study of Pain launched the second Global Day Against Pain, with a focus on Pain in Childhood. We hope this will be the start of an international emphasis on the importance of pain prevention and management in children.

References

1. United Nations. The Least Developed Countries Report 2002. New York: United Nations; 2002.
2. Bernstein S, Ryan WA, eds. The State of World Population 2003. United Nations Population Fund. Annapolis, MD: Prographics; 2003.
3. Neufeld V, MacLeod S, Tugwell P, Zakus D, Zarowsky C. The rich–poor gap in global health research: challenges for Canada. Can Med Assoc J 2001;164: 1158–1159.
4. Eland JM, Anderson JE. The experience of pain in children. In: Jacox A, ed. Pain: a Source Book for Nurses and Other Health Professionals. Boston: Little Brown; 1977:453–478.
5. Schechter NL, Allen DA, Hanson K. Status of pediatric pain control: a comparison of hospital analgesic usage in children and adults. Pediatrics 1986;77:11–15.
6. McCaffery M. Pain control: barriers to the use of available information. Cancer 1992;70:1438–1449.
7. Johnston CC, Gagnon AJ, Pepler CJ, Bourgault P. Pain in the emergency department with 1-wk follow-up of pain resolution. Pain Res Manag 2005;10:67–70.
8. Jacob E, Puntillo KA. Variability of analgesic practices for hospitalized children on different pediatric specialty units. J Pain Symptom Manage 2000;20:59–67.
9. Muirden N. Palliative care in Papua New Guinea: report of the International Association of Hospice and Palliative Care Travelling Fellowship. J Pain Palliat Care Pharmacother 2003;17:191–198.
10. Merriman A. Making drugs available. AIDS Action 1998;41:7.
11. McCarthy P, Chammas G, Wilimas J, Alaoui FM, Harif M. Managing children's cancer pain in Morocco. J Nurs Scholarsh 2004;36:11–15.
12. Williams DG, Hatch DJ, Howard RF. Codeine phosphate in paediatric medicine. Br J Anaesth 2001;86:413–421.
13. Pfefferbaum B, Adams J, Aceves J. The influence of culture on pain in Anglo and Hispanic children with cancer. J Am Acad Child Adolesc Psychiatry 1990;29: 642–647.
14. Harrison A. Childbirth in Kuwait: the experiences of three groups of Arab mothers. J Pain Symptom Manage 1991;8:466–475.
15. Maddocks I. Palliative care education in the developing countries. J Pain Palliat Care Pharmacother 2003;17:211–221.
16. Domino G, Regmi MP. Attitudes towards cancer: a cross-cultural comparison of Nepalese and US students. J Cross-Cult Psychol 1993;24:389–398.
17. Kodiath MF, Kodiath A. A comparative study of patients who experience chronic malignant pain in India and the United States. Cancer Nurs 1995;18:189–96.
18. Ali NS, Khalil HZ, Yousef W. A comparison of American and Egyptian cancer patients' attitudes and unmet needs. Cancer Nurs 1993;16:193–203.
19. Navon L. Voices from the world: Cultural views of cancer around the world. Cancer Nurs 1999;22:39–45.
20. Forgeron PA, Finley GA, Arnaout M. Pediatric pain prevalence and parents' attitudes at a cancer hospital in Jordan. J Pain Symptom Manage 2006;31.

21. Nolan T, Angos P, Cunha AJLA, et al. Quality of hospital care for seriously ill children in less-developed countries. Lancet 2001;357:106–110.
22. Nahata MC. Status of child health worldwide. Ann Pharmacother 1992;26:559–561.
23. Gaughan DM, Hughes MD, Seage GR, 3rd, et al. The prevalence of pain in pediatric human immunodeficiency virus/acquired immunodeficiency syndrome as reported by participants in the Pediatric Late Outcomes Study (PACTG 219). Pediatrics 2002;109:1144–1152.
24. Yaris N, Mandiracioglu A, Büyükpamukcu M. Childhood cancer in developing countries. Ped Hemat Oncol 2004;21:237–253.
25. Gbadoé AD, Atakouma DY, Akoli A, Assimadi, JK. Home care of vaso-occlusive crisis in sickle cell disease in Togo. Arch Pediatr 1999;6:958–961.
26. Chakravorty S, Newell K, Ramchandani J, et al. Sickle cell disease pain in London and the Caribbean. Arch Dis Child 2004;89:272, 273.
27. Rahman F, Rahman A, Linnan M, Giersing M, Shafinaz S. The magnitude of child injuries in Bangladesh: a major child health problem. Inj Control Saf Promot 2004;11:153–157.
28. Hofman K, Primack A, Keusch G, Hrynkow S. Addressing the growing burden of trauma and injury in low- and middle-income countries. Am J Public Health 2005;95:13–17
29. Ahuja RB, Bhattacharya S. Burns in the developing world and burn disasters. BMJ 2004;329:447–449.
30. Mabrouk A, Badawy AB, Sherif M. Kerosene stove as a cause of burns admitted to the Ain Shams burn unit. Burns 2000;26:474–477.
31. Panjeshahin MR, Lari AR, Talei AR, Shamsnia J, Alaghehbandan R. Epidemiology and mortality of burns in the South West of Iran. Burns 2001;27:219–226.
32. Ahuja RB, Bhattacharya S. An analysis of 11,196 burn admissions and evaluation of conservative management techniques. Burns 2002;28:555–561.
33. Walsh NE, Walsh WS. Rehabilitation of landmine victims—the ultimate challenge. Bull WHO 2003;81:665–670.
34. Coupland RM. The effect of weapons: defining superfluous injury and unnecessary suffering. Med Global Survival 1996;3:A1.
35. Lacoux PA, Crombie IK, Macrae WA. Pain in traumatic upper limb amputees in Sierra Leone. Pain 2002;99:309–312.
36. Franck LS, Cox S, Allen A, Winter I. Parental concern and distress about infant pain. Arch Dis Child Fetal Neonat Ed 2004;89:F71–F75.
37. Miles MS, Carter MC, Riddle I, Hennessey J, Eberly TW. The pediatric intensive care unit environment as a source of stress for parents. Matern Child Nurs J 1989;18:199–206.
38. Anand KJ, Sippell WG, Aynsley-Green A. Randomised trial of fentanyl anaesthesia in preterm babies undergoing surgery: effects on the stress response. Lancet 1987;1:62–66.
39. Ghooi RB, Ghooi SR. A mother in pain. Lancet 1998;352:1625.
40. Livingstone H. Pain relief in the developing world: the experience of Hospice Africa-Uganda. In: Rajagopal MR, Mazza D, Lipman AG, eds., Pain and Palliative

Care in the Developing World and Marginalized Populations. New York: Haworth Press; 2003;107–118.

41. Weissman DE, Haddox JD. Opioid pseudoaddiction-an iatrogenic syndrome. Pain 1989;36:363–366.

42. Joranson DE, Gilson AM, Ryan KM, Maurer MA. Availability of opioid analgesics for cancer pain relief in children. In: McGrath PJ, Finley GA, eds., Pediatric Pain: Biological and Social Context. Seattle, WA: IASP Press 2003;201–216.

43. Ghooi RB, Ghooi SR. Freedom from pain—a mirage or a possibility? Experience in attempts to change laws and practices in India. J Pain Palliat Care Pharmacother 2003;17:1–9.

44. DeSimone, GG. Palliative care in Argentina: perspectives from a country in crisis. J Pain Palliat Care Pharmacother 2003;17:23–43.

45. Ramsay S. Leading the way in African home-based palliative care. Lancet 2003;362: 1812, 1813.

46. Bollini P, Venkateswaran C, Sureshkumar K. Palliative care in Kerala, India: a model for resource-poor settings. Onkologie 2004;27:138–142.

47. Rajagopal MR, Venkateswaran C. Palliative care in India: successes and limitations. J Pain Palliat Care Pharmacother 2003;17:121–128.

48. Wenk R. Argentina: status of cancer pain and palliative care. J Pain Symptom Manage 1993;8:385–387.

49. Al-Hassan M, Alkhalil MS, Al-Ma'aitah R. Jordanian nurses' roles in the management of postoperative pain in the postanesthesia care unit. J Perianesth Nurs 1999;14:384–389.

50. Forgeron PA, Finley GA, Arnaout M. Introduction of a pediatric cancer pain program in Jordan [abstract]. World Congress on Pain, Sydney, Australia, August 22–26, 2005.

51. Morgan P. Some observations and lessons on capacity building. In: Maconick R, Morgan P, eds., Capacity Building Supported by the United Nations: Some Evaluations and Some Lessons. New York: United Nations; 1999.

52. Morgan P. An update on the performance monitoring of capacity development programs. What are we learning? Canadian International Development Agency Policy Branch. Paper presented at: DAC Informal Network on Institutional and Capacity Development; May 3–5th, 1999; Ottawa.

53. Wadsworth Y. What is participatory action research? Action Research International, 1998. Available at: http://www.scu.edu.au/schools/gcm/ar/ari/p-ywadsworth98.html1998. Accessed February 3, 2004.

54. Dick B. Action research: action and research. Action Research International, 2002. Available at: http://www.scu.edu.au/schools/gcm/ar/arp/aandr.html. Accessed August 10, 2005.

55. Muyinda H, Nakuya J, Whitworth AG, Pool R. Community sex education among adolescents in rural Uganda: utilizing indigenous institutions. AIDS Care 2004;16:69–79.

56. Aubel J, Toure I, Diagne M. Senegalese grandmothers promote improved maternal and child nutrition practices: the guardians of tradition are not averse to change. Soc Sci Med 2004;59:945–959.

57. Thassri J, Kala N, Chusintong L, Phongthanasarn J, Boonsrirat S, Jirojwong S. The development and evaluation of a health education programme for pregnant women in a regional hospital, southern Thailand. J Adv Nurs 2000;32:1450–1458.

58. World Health Organization. Cancer Pain Relief and Palliative Care in Children. Geneva; WHO, 1980.

59. Jabbour S. Health and development in the Arab world: which way forward? BMJ 2003;326:1141–1143.

60. Garner P, Meremikwu M, Volmink J, Xu Q, Smith H. Putting evidence into practice: how middle and low income countries "get it together." BMJ 2004;329:1036–1039.

61. Neufeld V. Introduction presented at: First Summer Institute for "New" Global Health Researchers; Canadian Coalition for Global Health Research; July 10–15, 2004; hosted by International Health Office, Dalhousie University, Halifax, Nova Scotia, Canada.

9

Knowledge Translation and Pain Management

Shannon Scott-Findlay and Carole A. Estabrooks

Summary

Over the last few decades, there has been substantial growth in pediatric pain research, yet children continue to endure pain despite this well-established body of evidence. Assessing, treating, and managing pain in children is complex because of the developmental issues involved in assessing and understanding the child's pain, the nature and the structure of health care professionals' work, the immense and varied influences on health care professionals' decisions, the heuristics or mental shortcuts that health care professionals use to cope in high-velocity environments overloaded with information, the added challenges with children with developmental delays, and a host of personal attitudes and beliefs about pain. These factors and others contribute to poor pain management in children. We believe, however, that the core challenge to improving pediatric pain management is knowledge translation. Rather than an issue of knowledge deficit or lack of research (although these are nontrivial), we argue that the core issue is a failure to put what we already know to use. In this chapter, we discuss knowledge translation challenges in relation to pediatric pain management and to offer possible solutions to closing the gap between science and practice.

Key Words: Knowledge transfer; knowledge translation; pain management; research utilization.

1. Introduction

Over the last few decades, there has been substantial growth in pediatric pain research. This research has led to improved techniques to assess pain in children, an increased repertoire of treatment approaches, and an increased theoretical understanding of children's pain. However, despite advances in science, pain in neonates, infants, and children remains inadequately managed (*1–3*).

Clinical practice, unfortunately, does not always reflect the latest research. In the United States, Sung (*4*) stressed that the translation of basic scientific knowledge into clinical studies and the translation of clinical studies into improvements

From: *Bringing Pain Relief to Children: Treatment Approaches*
Edited by: G. A. Finley, P. J. McGrath, and C. T. Chambers © Humana Press Inc., Totowa, NJ

in health care practices are two major obstacles or translational blocks in the health care system. Sung suggested that the risk run by not attending to these obstacles is that scientific discoveries will fail to become translated into tangible human benefits; this is the issue that we are seeing with pediatric pain research. Despite all of the research on pediatric pain, children continue to suffer uncontrolled pain. To illustrate the magnitude of this lack of transfer, studies in the United States and the Netherlands suggested that 30–40% of patients do not receive care that complies with current research evidence, and 20–25% of the care provided is not needed and may be potentially harmful *(5,6)*.

The detrimental consequences of inadequate pediatric pain management are being uncovered in a rapidly expanding body of research. This body of research highlights the physiological, anatomical, and behavioral effects of pain. For example, neonates who have experienced strong, enduring pain or repeated types of noxious stimulation may develop chronic pain *(7)* and altered future pain perceptions *(8)*. Repeated exposure to noxious stimulation *(9)* may cause molecular alterations in the experience of pain. Untreated pain in infants may result in marked increases in heart rates and blood pressure, increased chemical and hormone release, and breakdown of fat and carbohydrate stores *(10,11)*. Untreated pain may also result in psychosocial problems, cognitive deficits, poor motor performance, and a rise in somatic complaints of unknown origin *(12)*. Some children who have experienced very painful procedures may go on to experience long-term sequelae that resemble posttraumatic stress syndrome, with physical symptoms, such as stomachaches and bad dreams *(12)*. And finally, unresolved pediatric pain is associated with rehospitalization and an increase in the utilization of health services *(13)*.

The consequences of experiencing pain as neonates, infants, or children are well recognized. This research base ought to compel clinicians to use pediatric pain research when making decisions about treating children's pain. However, we generally recognize—indeed, lament—the reality that clinicians do not base their pain management practices on sound scientific evidence, and that children still suffer in pain. This gap between research and practice, although not unique to the field of pain management, is particularly perplexing in what would seem on first examination to be an area with optimum implementation of research.

Assessing, treating, and managing pain in children is complex. Managing pain in children is challenging because of the developmental issues in assessing and understanding the child's pain, the nature and the structure of health care professionals' work, the immense and varied influences on health care professionals' decisions, the heuristics or mental shortcuts that health care professionals use to cope in high-velocity environments overloaded with information, the added challenges with children with developmental delays, and a host of personal attitudes and beliefs about pain. These factors and others contribute to poor pain management in children. We believe, however, that the core challenge to improving pediatric pain management is a knowledge translation challenge. Rather than an issue of knowledge deficit or lack of research (although these are nontrivial), we argue that the core issue is failure to put what we already know to use.

The purpose of this chapter is to discuss knowledge translation challenges in relation to pediatric pain management and to offer possible solutions to closing the gap between science and practice. The chapter is organized as follows:

1. The problem.
2. Locating the knowledge translation field.
3. Definition and clarification of knowledge translation.
4. What we know from existing knowledge translation research.
5. The nature and sources of practice knowledge and why it matters.
6. Possible solutions.
7. Conclusions.

2. What Is the Problem?

We perceive that scholars within the pediatric pain community may view the existence of inadequate pediatric pain management as a primarily knowledge deficit problem, whether that deficit is in the actual volume of available research or in clinician's awareness of that research. We see repeated calls for increasing the amount of pediatric pain research; often, they present in the form of "if we only knew more" then children would not be suffering in pain *(14)*. As recent as the joint scientific meeting of the American Pain Society and the Canadian Pain Society *(15)*, one of the major priorities was increasing the amount of research into pediatric pain. We believe that although both new science about pediatric pain and increased clinician knowledge about pain management are important, neither increasing pediatric pain research nor deploying strategies aimed at increasing clinician knowledge—alone or together—will solve the challenges of pediatric pain management. We know from previous work that even if clinicians have adequate knowledge they do not automatically use it. Such approaches are rooted in traditional science push and dissemination models of knowledge translation *(16)*.

An examination of Rogers's classic innovation diffusion theory illustrates the complexity of challenges of diffusing innovations *(19)*. We argue that although there are important differences between innovations and research, they are sufficiently similar to warrant serious consideration of Rogers's work. He and others *(17)* offered numerous examples dating back many decades that illustrate the lengthy periods of time it takes from the development of an innovation to its use.

An example commonly used is that of the use of citrus juice for the prevention of scurvy. In the 15th and 16th centuries, scurvy was the most significant cause of death on long sea voyages. In 1601, James Lancaster, an English sea captain, tested the effectiveness of citrus juice in preventing scurvy on four ships. The men on the ship that received the citrus juice stayed relatively healthy, yet this was not the case with the three control ships. The effectiveness of citrus juice in preventing scurvy seemed clear. However, despite these convincing results, it took 264 years and further investigations and reinvention of Lancaster's initial idea before citrus juice was widely accepted as a scurvy prevention *(18,19)*. This example, although extreme, illustrates the frustratingly slow rate at which many innovations diffuse.

In the innovation of the diffusion process, individuals (or groups) pass first from knowledge of an innovation to forming an attitude toward the innovation, to a decision to adopt or reject it, to implementation and use of the new idea, and to confirmation of the decision *(19)*. Five steps constitute the process: (1) knowledge, (2) persuasion, (3) decision, (4) implementation, and (5) confirmation. It is obvious that simply producing new knowledge will not attend to the research-practice gap; the other four steps needed to be considered. Until recently, many believed that simply giving people information will cause them to change their behavior. However, we now know that knowledge only is inadequate.

A study in *Nursing Research* illustrated that, even if health care professionals have the knowledge, they may not use it. In this study, Stastny and colleagues *(20)* studied nursery nurses' knowledge about placing infants in the supine position potentially to decrease the risk of sudden infant death syndrome. Their results showed that although 72% of nursery staff knew that the supine position was the most appropriate for lowering the risk of sudden infant death, only 30% of staff actually placed newborns in that position. The research by Stastny and colleagues demonstrates that health care professionals' behavior does not change on the basis of knowledge alone.

3. Locating the Knowledge Translation Field

Some 25 years ago, Larsen *(21)* described an unresolved "terminological tangle" in the knowledge utilization and related fields. Throughout this chapter, we use the term *knowledge translation* to refer to the large interdisciplinary field of study encompassing knowledge translation, knowledge mobilization, innovation diffusion, technology transfer, research dissemination, research utilization, evidence-based medicine, evidence-based decision making, and so on. In nursing (and in social work), the field is often referred to as *research utilization*. We are most familiar with and often use the following terms interchangeably: knowledge translation, knowledge utilization, and research utilization. However, caution must be used because these are not in fact synonymous terms.

In the early 1990s, we witnessed the emergence of evidence-based medicine *(22)* and subsequent more general calls for the adoption of an evidence-based decision-making culture in the health care system *(23,24)*. The emergence of evidence-based medicine is a contemporary attempt to root practice and policy decisions in science. Nursing has a longer tradition in the broad knowledge translation area, specifically in the narrower field of research utilization, dating from the 1970s *(25,26)*. In nursing, there is widespread agreement that the large Conduct and Utilization of Research in Nursing project *(27,28)* of the 1970s is the common demarcation of nursing efforts in this field. In related health disciplines, such as physiotherapy, occupational therapy, and dentistry, the advent of identifiable activity in this field is more recent *(29)*.

In Canada, the Canadian Institutes of Health Research adopted the term *knowledge translation*, defining it as "the exchange, synthesis and ethically-sound application of knowledge—within a complex system of interactions among researchers and users—to accelerate the capture of the benefits of research for Canadians through improved health, more effective services and products, and a strengthened health care system" *(30)*.

4. What Is Knowledge Translation?

The goal of knowledge translation activities is to increase the use of relevant knowledge, commonly research, among clinicians, managers, administrators, and policy makers. Knowledge translation is a social process—a process in which research is considered among other things, personal preferences, professional group norms, and the values of the organization or setting in which the decision is made. It involves directing time and energy along at least three key dimensions: audience, message, and delivery. The knowledge must be tailored to the audience receiving it and be congruent with their values; the message must be delivered in a manner that resonates with the intended audience. Knowledge translation problems are complex because they involve behavior change among providers working in complex and high-velocity health care organizations. Such behavior change is optimally rooted in an ability to influence decision-making behaviors to fit with the new knowledge and the system of care delivery and not solely with changing behavior in the absence of decision-making changes (i.e., in an exclusively protocol-driven approach).

Pediatric health care professionals who have responsibilities for managing children's pain work within these complex organizational structures and have competing demands from multiple stakeholders (e.g., supervisors, colleagues, students, patients, families, drug representatives, etc.). These groups of people all influence the clinicians' decision making. If we assume that the primary problem is the need to fill a knowledge deficit or to bring more research on pain management to providers' awareness, then the influence of these groups of people is not as important. Rather, the provider would be rational (free from influences) and consider only objective research evidence. However, many clinicians do not have sophisticated research assessment skills that enable them to assess the quality of the research thoroughly *(31)*. Even if a clinician has relatively up-to-date knowledge of the latest developments in pediatric pain research, they may not have the time, skills, organizational understanding, or authority to change practices.

5. What Does Knowledge Translation Science Tell Us?

The determinants of research utilization are often separated into the broad areas of evidence, individuals, organizations, and sometimes policy or broader societal determinants. Of most relevance to this chapter are the individual and organizational categories. Pain management is a unique area in the knowledge translation field, largely because it has reasonably robust evidence. Knowledge specific to the evidence is usually focused on the characteristics of evidence after it is packaged for an audience. Current wisdom is that for an innovation (e.g., a pain protocol) to be optimal, it would have the following characteristics: relative advantage, compatibility, complexity, trialability, and observability *(32,33)*. In addition, the extent to which providers can reinvent or modify the innovation to suit their circumstances is thought to aid in the usability of research *(32,34)*. Rather than address evidence characteristics in depth in this chapter, Lemieux-Charles and Barnsley *(35)* recently provided an in-depth treatment of innovation diffusion in health care, including a discussion of characteristics of the evidence.

5.1. Individual Determinants

Individual determinants of research use include those factors generally accepted to reside in the individual provider and hence are amenable to interventions targeted at changing or influencing individual behavior as opposed to changing the context. We have argued elsewhere for a shift from the study of individual determinants to more study of context *(29,36)*. We argue here that the challenges of knowledge translation in pediatric pain management commonly manifest themselves in decision-making processes and in the attitudes, beliefs, and values that individuals hold about pediatric pain and its management and that addressing these elements of the knowledge translation challenge in pain management requires a relatively balanced approach to the study of individual and contextual determinants.

5.1.1. General Considerations

Rogers *(19)* grouped adopter characteristics into three categories: (1) socio-economic characteristics (education, social status, income, social mobility, literacy, age, favorable attitude toward borrowing money, etc.); (2) personality variables (empathy, dogmatism, ability to deal with abstractions, rationality, intelligence, positive change attitude, ability to cope with uncertainty, favorable attitude toward education, optimism/fatalism, high levels of achievement motivation); and (3) communication behavior (social participation, interconnected social systems, cosmopoliteness, change agent contact, contact with interpersonal communication channels, knowledge of innovations, high levels of opinion leadership, and existence as part of highly interconnected systems).

Writing many years ago, Jacoby *(37)* found a positive association between low levels of dogmatism and innovative behavior. He described dogmatism as a functional characteristic in that the "more persistently anxious or threatened the individual, the more he maintains a closed mind." It is probably closely related to resistance to change and conservatism and its corollaries open-mindedness or cognitive flexibility. Mohr *(38)* suggested a conservatism–liberalism continuum, with higher levels of conservatism associated with less innovation adoption. The ability to cope with uncertainty and risk was cited by Kimberly *(39)*, Rogers *(40)*, and Warner *(41)* as important to successful innovation.

Scott and Bruce *(42)* identified problem-solving style (i.e., intuitive vs systematic) as an important variable in influencing innovation. Morrow-Bradley and Elliott *(43)*, studying psychologists, reported that "the strongest, most consistent correlate of research utilization was theoretical orientation; behavioral (including cognitive) therapists reported finding therapy research more useful, whereas dynamic therapists found it less useful." Cohen et al. *(44)* supported this idea. The concept of a theoretical orientation influencing research utilization is essentially unexplored in the health sciences.

5.1.2. Nursing

We completed a systematic review examining individual determinants that influence research use in nursing. We examined published articles with authors who had studied the influence of individual factors on the research utilization behaviors of nurses *(45)*. Six categories of potential individual determinants were identified: beliefs and attitudes, involvement in research activities, information seeking, professional characteristics, education, and other socioeconomic factors. Methodological problems (e.g., sampling, measurement, etc.) surfaced in all of the studies, and except for a positive attitude to research, we were unable to assert any of the measured individual determinants as influencing research use. We concluded that this area of study was too underdeveloped among health professionals, specifically nurses, to offer clear directions. However, it is clear that, in nursing at least, many of what might be construed as relevant factors have not been studied. For example, a genuinely individual set of determinants is more likely to include such psychological variables as cognitive flexibility and open-mindedness; however, to date, these categories of variables have been largely absent, at least from nursing studies. Instead, individual determinants have included such variables as educational level, autonomy (more likely a function of the organization than the individual), and so forth.

5.1.3. Medicine

In the medical literature, scholars have advocated several general approaches to knowledge translation or, as it is more often described, research implementation. These include the development and dissemination of clinical practice guidelines *(46,47)*, computerized decision support systems *(48,49)*, continuous quality improvement *(50)*, and continuing medical education *(51,52)*. The Cochrane Effective Practice and Organization of Care group has conducted systematic reviews *(53–55)* to assess the effectiveness of these broad strategies. These reviews suggested that the effects of interventions tend to fall into three groups. First are the interventions that are consistently effective in promoting behavioral change: outreach visits, reminders, and interactive educational materials. Second, there are interventions that have variable effectiveness: audit and feedback, the use of local opinion leaders, and local consensus processes. Finally, there are interventions that have minimal effect on practitioner behavior change: educational materials and didactic educational sessions *(53)*.

Generally, systematic reviews of the effectiveness of interventions for modifying physician provider behavior have concluded that there are no guaranteed approaches for ensuring practitioner behavior change, that most interventions are effective under particular conditions, and no interventions are effective under all circumstances or in all contexts *(52,53,56–58)*. Oxman and colleagues *(52)* review highlights the reality that there are no "magic bullets" for improving the quality of health care, but rather there is a range of interventions that can be used that may lead to changes in clinician behavior.

Some of the frequently studied interventions tested to change clinician behavior are educational material, conferences, outreach visits, local opinion leaders, audit and feedback, reminder systems (computerized or paper), and local consensus approaches. It is noteworthy that 80% of existing interventions used in implementation research focus on changing individual behavior *(59)* as compared with changing the systems in which the practitioners work. The work of Solberg *(60)* suggested that, because of the challenges inherent in changing individual behavior, perhaps a more productive solution is to focus on creating systems or clinical environments that support the desired behavior (in this case, using research in practice).

There has been debate in the medical literature on the effectiveness of multiple interventions. Multiple interventions are defined as the co-occurrence of two or more interventions at one time. Oxman and colleagues *(52)* argued that when interventions are used in combination, the effects may be significant. Grimshaw and colleagues *(59)*, the Royal Society of Medicine *(56)*, and Gross and colleagues

(61) also supported multifaceted interventions. However, more recent work by Grimshaw and colleagues *(62)* exploring the effectiveness of different guideline dissemination and implementation strategies found no relationship between the number of interventions and the effects of multifaceted interventions. Grimshaw and Eccles *(63)* added weight to this finding by suggesting that multifaceted interventions may not be more effective than single interventions. There is currently insufficient evidence regarding whether multifaceted interventions are more effective than single interventions. The inconsistency of the notion of single vs multifaceted interventions indicates that more research is needed into this aspect of knowledge transfer.

There is a developing, but as yet inadequate, base of evidence to guide the development of implementation strategies to enhance the use of research in practice. Many of the current approaches to research implementation in clinical practice are based on the researchers' beliefs, such as "I think that this will work," rather than basing the intervention on the research evidence or emerging theory *(64)*. Strategies to implement research need to be based on evidence; in other words, we require evidence-based implementation *(64)*. In many cases, it is unclear from study reports why particular interventions are chosen, and as a result, we do not know whether the interventions can be generalized to other contexts or providers *(63)*. The Medical Research Council in the United Kingdom developed a framework for the development and evaluation of interventions to improve health outcomes *(65)*. This framework advocates the development of the theoretical basis for interventions.

5.1.4. Lessons From Health Promotion

A look at the health promotion literature illustrates the challenge of making and maintaining behavior change. For instance, Perri *(66)* demonstrated relapse rates of nearly 80% for lifestyle modifications such as weight loss and physical activity. However, Grimshaw and colleagues *(62)* suggested that it is possible to change health care providers' behavior. They argued that small-to-moderate improvements in providers' care can be actualized through reminders, educational materials, audit and feedback, and multifaceted interventions. Continuing to look at the health promotion literature for insight, we know that strategies most likely to succeed are ones based on clearly defining the behavior to be changed and on an understanding of the environmental context *(67)*.

The necessity for thoroughly understanding the context prior to undertaking any change was echoed by Effective Health Care *(56)*, which stated that the reasons for explaining why research-based recommendations are not routinely adopted into practice are multifaceted. In spite of this, they advocated prior to the implementation of any research-based recommendation, such as a clinical guideline, that a period of "information and diagnostic analysis" be first completed. The initial analysis of the context would likely involve:

1) identification of all groups involved in, affected by or influencing the proposed change(s), 2) assessment of the characteristics of the proposed change that might influence its adoption, 3) assessment of the preparedness of the health professionals to change and other potentially relevant internal factors within the target group, 4) identification of potential external barriers to change, and 5) identification of likely enabling factors, including resources and skills.

The information from the diagnostic analysis would inform the development of an appropriate implementation strategy.

5.1.5. Guideline Implementation

Guidelines have been touted as a useful approach to transfer knowledge *(47)*. Guidelines are "systematically developed statements to assist practitioners' and patients' decisions about the appropriate care for specified clinical outcomes" *(68)*. However, their mere existence does not mean that they will be used in clinical practice. Standards for the development and evaluation of guidelines have been created *(69,70)*. From previous investigations, we do know that guidelines are more likely to be valid if they have been developed from meta-analysis and have been developed by national organizations with multidisciplinary representation *(71)*.

There has been discussion regarding the most appropriate medium for guideline implementation. The media for implementing guidelines are commonly hard copy or computer mediated. Jousimaa and colleagues *(72)*, however, compared the effects of computer vs paper-based guidelines on recently qualified physicians and found no difference in their use; they suggested that the method of presenting guidelines does not significantly influence guideline use or the guideline's impact on decisions. However, computer-generated guidelines do offer other advantages: they are easier to update, have lower production costs compared with paper-based material, offer more opportunities to link with other technologies, and the electronic medium facilitates monitoring the usage of the guidelines. Yet, the use of computer-generated guidelines demands that clinicians have access and a level of comfort with the technology.

5.1.6. Values, Attitudes, and Beliefs

Health care professionals, in addition to using heuristics to cope in complex environments in which they are facing large amounts of information, also bring to bear beliefs and attitudes about pediatric pain management. A complex interaction of interests, beliefs, and ideologies create the emergence of values *(73)*. Inadequate pediatric pain management affects the individual child experiencing the pain, the child's family, as well as the health care workers involved in their care. In spite of all that we do know about pediatric pain management, many people still hold myths and misconceptions about pediatric pain. For example, some believe that young children do not experience pain because of neurological immaturity *(74)*. However, we know from research that by 30 weeks' gestation the pain pathways and cortical and subcortical centers necessary for pain perception are developed *(75)*. Therefore, children do experience pain, and they can remember pain.

Despite all of the pediatric research to date, myths still abound. Myths, such as opioids are addictive in therapeutic doses, pain builds character, and children will tell you if they are in pain, are still persistent *(74)*. If people hold these values about pain, then it is difficult to get them to change their attitudes and beliefs. As Lomas *(73)* argued, values are at the core of whether and how we are able to change decision-making processes in complex organizations. So, although they pose significant challenges to us, those values that we can consider beliefs (as opposed to core ideological values) are of considerable importance in planning successful strategies that facilitate research uptake in practice.

5.2. The Organization

At the organizational level, we discuss the challenges that complex organizational structures present when individuals or groups attempt to implement research. Traditionally, new research has been disseminated by peer-reviewed journals and continuing education programs *(63)*; however, the effectiveness of these passive strategies has been called into question. Using research in practice demands change at several levels, including the organizational level and the larger system level *(76)*. Consequently, different theory is needed at these different levels. For instance, at the individual level, theory drawn from cognitive psychology may be relevant and inform individual practice change, whereas organizational and system theory have utility when considering the organization.

As we discuss organizational theory relevant to knowledge translation, we rely heavily on earlier work by Estabrooks *(36)*. Throughout history, a number of issues considered to have an impact on innovation adoption have been examined, although comparatively few studies have been documented that focused particularly on the influence of these or related factors on research or knowledge utilization. The organizational factors with influence on innovation adoption that have been customarily examined—usually by those outside the realm of nursing—include "organizational complexity, centralization, size, presence of a research champion, traditionalism, organizational slack, time, access to and amount of resources, professional autonomy and organizational support" *(36)*.

5.2.1. Organizational Complexity

In organizational studies completed separately, Damanpour *(77)*, Meyer and Goes *(78)*, Mohr *(38)*, and Orlandi *(79)* examined organizational *complexity*, which is generally considered to consist of functional differentiation, specialization, and professionalism *(80)*. Damanpour *(81)* established in a meta-analysis that in organizations these factors are normally positively linked with innovation diffusion.

5.2.2. Centralization

Generally, investigators hold that *centralization* of authority and decision making inhibits innovative thinking and behavior. This perspective has been studied by Kimberly *(82)*, Kimberly and Evanisko *(83)*, and Moch and Morse *(84)*, who reported that indeed the presence of centralization of authority and decision making exerts a negative effect on the adoption of innovations *(81)*.

5.2.3. Organizational Size

Organizational size can be construed as a positive influence on the adoption of innovations; that is, the larger the organization is, the more adoption of innovations there will be *(38,78,80,83–86)*. In Mohr's *(38)* study of health units, he drew attention to the fact that size, most likely, indicates other variables, such as presence of motivation, obstacles, and resources. While Rogers *(19)* concurred, he suggested that, although size is most likely repeatedly investigated because it is simple to measure and relatively precise, researchers must search to discover the underlying structure of size rather than studying this substitute variable. In nursing, Varcoe and Hilton *(87)* published findings that indicated organizational support and expectations about research use varied in accordance to size, whereas Brett *(88,89)* published findings that indicated there is "no relationship between size of the hospital and adoption of innovations by nurses" *(36)*.

5.2.4. Innovation (or Research) Champions

Transferring knowledge involves the movement of knowledge from one place or group of people to another. It is an implicit, often tenuous, act and often requires facilitation by a catalyst. To this point, most transfer activity has focused on "push" models, with researchers disseminating their research and encouraging its use. A more constructive approach that focuses on collaborative problem-solving relationships between researchers and decision makers involves cultivating linkages between decision makers and researchers and results in mutual learning. In this process, intermediaries are key. These intermediaries bring researchers and decision makers together, facilitating their interaction so that they are able to understand better each other's goals and professional cultures, to influence each other's work, to forge new partnerships, and to use research-based evidence. This process requires people who can link the world of academia with the world of decision makers, policy setters, and clinicians.

Investigators have shown a positive influence on the adoption of innovations and the utilization of research through the use of an innovation or research champion *(90–93)*. In the knowledge translation literature, a host of monikers have been used to describe the role of intermediaries in the transference of research into practice, roles such as facilitators, knowledge brokers, champions, linking agents, opinion leaders, and change agents. The emergence of these roles is an obvious indication that passive dissemination is inadequate. Rather, the translation of research into practice requires interpersonal contact to facilitate the likelihood of behavioral change.

However, Thompson and colleagues *(94)*, through a critical analysis of the intermediary literature, suggested that there is inconsistency in the use of these concepts. They further pointed out that these role descriptors may be variations of the same phenomena.

Although the judicious use of research champions (and other intermediary roles) is clearly important, this conceptual inconsistency poses challenges when comparing intervention work in the knowledge translation literature.

5.2.5. Traditionalism

Relatively little has been written about traditionalism. Mohr *(38)* and Mohr and Downs *(95)* mentioned traditionalism from the perspective that the less traditional an organization is, the more predisposed the organization would be to innovate. Likewise, in their discussion of organizational climate, Scott and Bruce *(42)* inferred that more creative organizations, that is, less traditional organizations, facilitate more innovation. Last, Rogers *(19)* indicated that innovative organizations are more creative and flexible, that is, less traditional.

5.2.6. Organizational Slack

Organizational slack can be defined as uncommitted resources in the system *(19,38,80–82,96,97)*. Investigators believe that within organizations with a higher degree of slack, more innovation occurs. Health care providers seldom experience the advantage of slack in a similar way that private sector employees have. For example, "the structural constraints that operate on the delivery of patient care in hospitals and other health organizations have not resulted in slack being experienced at the point of care delivery" *(36)*.

5.2.7. Time

In the nursing literature, we see lack of time identified repeatedly as exerting an unfavorable influence on research use *(98–105)*. Little has been written to clarify what is meant by the notion of *time* to nurses in general or "more specifically within the context of research utilization" *(36)*. From personal experience, in our work we see *busyness* and *interruptedness** as dimensions of this at best loosely conceived construct of time.

5.2.8. Access to Research and Resources

Another factor important to the utilization of research in nursing consistently identified is access to research and resources, which includes findings, studies, libraries, and other sources *(98,100,105,106)*. Other than the institutional paper-based research library, additional research sources thus far have not received a great deal of interest in the research utilization literature. As technologies make their way into workplaces (i.e., the Internet), this lack of attention is anticipated to change. However, aspects of access to research and resources that have been investigated include accessible research facilities and information accessibility at work *(99,107,108)*, research knowledge and research teams *(104,109)*, presence at conferences, and accessibility of research journal clubs *(36,110)*.

5.2.9. Professional Autonomy

Regarding organizational variables believed to have an impact on research utilization behaviors of nurses, some support has been given to professional autonomy *(98,101,105,111)*. However, the aforementioned investigators were ambiguous regarding whether they were dealing with organizational, professional, or individual autonomy. Because professional autonomy has been seldom studied and considering its importance in other connected areas of work, professional autonomy's significance may be undervalued *(112–114)*.

5.2.10. Support

Within the framework of nurses' workplaces, several kinds of support have been recognized as significant to the use of research. These include peer support *(100)*; support of nursing leaders/administration *(98,100,101,115)*; support of other members of the health care team, such as physicians, physiotherapists, etc. *(101,116)*; a supportive infrastructure for nursing research *(103,106)*; and administrative support expressed in both material and less-tangible ways *(36,106,117–119)*.

**Busyness* has both subjective and objective aspects. It is an individual perception of internalized pressure created by a situation in which there is a shortage of time to accomplish valued work and often results in a reduced energy level. Objectively, it is characterized by much action or motion. Busyness is influenced by factors such as workload, coping ability, and environmental complexity (Thompson D, O'Leary K, Scott-Findlay S, Jensen E, and Estabrooks C, 2005, unpublished data). *Interruptedness* describes the activity of being interrupted.

5.2.11. Organizational Context and Organizational Culture

Increasingly, context (sometimes described as culture) is regarded as significant in influencing the use of research in clinical practice *(98,106,120,121)*. We see a marked shift in efforts to understand its significance. Though context (or culture) has been pointed to as significant, little empirical work has been done to understand the process through which it exerts its influence. So, although nursing scholars have been successful in identifying features that influence research use, more sophisticated analytic work has not been completed, such as the development of models that demonstrate how the identified features interact and work. Specifically, until this time, scholars have been unable to provide specific detail regarding how and why the organizational context is important.

Some of the most significant conceptual work in nursing about the influence of context on the utilization of research came from Kitson and colleagues *(121–123)*. They proposed that successful research use is a function of the interplay of three core elements: evidence, facilitation, and context. Within this theoretical work, context is more traditionally conceptualized as the physical environment, where the prevailing culture is a component of the context. In our research, we have adopted both an emerging understanding of culture that asserts that organizations *are* cultures *(124–130)* and a view that culture is a transformable characteristic within a context *(130)*. We find both perspectives useful but suspect that the emerging organization as culture view, which draws heavily on organizational science theory, particularly the work of Schein *(131)* and Hatch *(127,128,132)*, may optimistically yield some explanatory rationale for culture's role in knowledge translation.

5.2.12. Implications: Mixed Models

From existing research, it is challenging to extract concrete conclusions regarding the effect of the organizational context. Nonetheless, results thus far imply that organizational variables and nursing unit practices wield strong influences on research utilization. Organizational context could be the critical factor in leveraging individual determinants to exert more impact *(36)*. Consequently, to study the influences on research utilization, researchers in the field must implement a more "ecological" approach by mixed models that put together individual, unit, organizational, and regional levels of analysis. It is vital to build greater focus on organizational models of research utilization. We now realize that organizations exercise considerable influences on both patient and nurse outcomes *(133,134)*.

5.2.13. Communities of Practice

When looking at factors influencing how nurses manage their practice, we are increasingly conscious of the significant role that groups and their interactions play. For example, most nursing knowledge is not presented nor does it exist as "discrete 'bits' of knowledge that are written down and acquired by reading" *(36)*. Rather, nursing knowledge presents, is developed in, and is transmitted via numerous smaller, often intersecting, "communities of practice." This idea of communities of practice, initially originating in the field of education *(135,136)*, has not, however, been applied seriously in the organizational or knowledge utilization literature. Nevertheless, this idea does fit well with what nurses tend to encounter in their working lives and is congruent with trends emerging in some of our data. Researchers are discovering that, regarding both the production and transfer of knowledge, people do not learn in isolation, but the development of community is crucial.

When applied to nursing, the theory of communities of practice implies that nurses interact with the people with whom they work and practice creatively with the resources and tools that are easily accessible. Essentially, what this means is that to get their jobs done, nurses do not always act in prescribed or predictable ways but rather use the resources that they have at hand. According to Lave and Wenger *(135)*, it is throughout this negotiation of what does and does not work that nurses jointly create a community of practice. Nurses "green" to the nursing unit need to understand the way things are done on this unit; if successful, they may eventually become full members of this small community of practice *(36)*.

Increasingly, we are mindful that nurses depend more on knowledge produced within their communities of practice than on knowledge produced from research. A significant concept underpinning communities of practice is that learning is social. The preceptor/new nurse relationship, for instance, can be an important way to transfer knowledge concerning both unit-based norms and professional knowledge. In 1991, Lave and Wenger described this action of advancing into full membership as "the learning of knowledgeable skills" *(135)*.

6. Ongoing Research

Our research program, the Knowledge Utilization Studies Program at the University of Alberta (http://www.ualberta.ca/~kusp), addresses the need for a theoretical basis for interventions. Theory development is one of the central objectives of this research program. We have a particular focus on the context in which providers practice and the interaction of multiple levels of decision making in complex organizations. One of the areas of study in our unit relevant to the present chapter is the set of findings from what we describe as the Research Utilization Studies described in the sections that follow.

6.1. Research Utilization Studies

The multicenter Research Utilization Studies are ethnographic case study projects in which we examined the factors influencing nurses' research utilization behaviors. Data were collected between 1999 and 2003. These projects were done by a multidisciplinary group of researchers from the Universities of Alberta and Toronto and were funded by the Canadian Institute for Health Research and Alberta Heritage Foundation for Medical Research. The first project, Determinants of Research Utilization: Pain Management in Adults, centered on pain management in adults and was carried out between 1999 and 2002. The second project, The Determinants of Research Utilization: Pain Management in Infants and Children, concentrated on pain management in infants and children between 2000 and 2003.

Cases in these studies totaled seven: five pediatric and two adult acute care units. Data were gathered throughout a 6-month phase of fieldwork at each nursing unit. The units were located in four tertiary-level university-affiliated hospitals. We used participant observation, interviews, and focus groups to collect qualitative data. Patients, families, nurses, other health practitioners involved in pain management, unit managers, program managers, and other administrative personnel were interviewed. Supplementary sources of data included notes taken while present at pertinent unit activities (e.g., reports between shifts and unit meetings that concentrated on care planning), unit documents (e.g., mission and policy statements), as well as documents connected to standards of care.

Quantitative data collected included a number of pain scales administered to patients. Data collected from nurses included measures of research utilization, critical thinking dispositions, environmental complexity, and organizational culture. Demographic, organizational structure, and nursing skill mix data were also collected.

At the nursing unit level, factors influencing research utilization by nurses were characteristics of the local environment, characteristics of the larger organizational context, and of particular note, leadership style on the patient care unit. We observed that both the use of research and the manner in which this use was expressed varied among professions. Physicians, for example, demonstrated research use in what we would consider a fairly classic manner: verbally in rounds using scientific language. The use of research by nurses, on the other hand, was embedded in everyday actions and conversations and therefore difficult to recognize as explicit research use. Within the nursing profession, there are variations in the use of research and the expression of that use, depending on the role and position of the nurse. Our findings suggested that nurses also rely heavily on tacit sources of knowledge. In these studies, nurses preferred "interactions in the workplace as sources of practice knowledge, in particular, but not restricted to, peer-to-peer interactions and exchanges" *(137)*.

Traditional accounts in the nursing literature indicate that because of a lack of time, nurses do not use research. However, we could not support this claim in our data. Our findings suggested that high workloads as such may not be an important barrier for research use. In fact, drawing on some theory from the organizational sciences *(138,139)* higher workloads may actually be associated with higher than predicted levels of research use. Our findings pointed to possible interventions or strategies to increase the uptake and use of research by nurses and other health care practitioners.

6.2. Sources of Knowledge

Several studies reporting sources of practice knowledge used by nurses are published; all used survey methods *(140–142)*. We located no studies that asked clinicians themselves to describe and categorize the kinds of knowledge needed to practice or any that attempted to understand how clinicians privilege various knowledge sources. Drawing on individual and card sort interviews, as well as participant observations, in the research utilization studies described above, we identified nurses' sources of practice knowledge. Our findings suggested that nurses categorize their sources of practice knowledge into four broad group-ings: social interactions, experiential knowledge, documents, and *a priori* knowledge *(143)*. Experiential knowledge and knowledge produced in and shared via interactions were the most commonly identified sources. In addition, the choice of knowledge source is influenced by factors such as trust, hierarchy, question specificity, time, and knowledge presentation style *(144)*. This work suggested that, rather than continue with historically preferred interventions to increase research use (e.g., training in critical appraisal), more productive approaches will be found in developing interventions that complement rather than ignore existing sources of practice knowledge, sources that we argue exist for legitimate reasons and not because nurses in this case are somehow deficient in their abilities to consume and apply the findings of scientific reports.

6.3. Heuristics in Nursing

Heuristics are cognitive shortcuts that help people make decisions. These cognitive shortcuts are considered a component of the decision-making litera-ture. In this chapter, we are not discussing the decision-making literature in health care *(145,146)*; rather, we are simply highlighting how our ongoing work on health care professionals' use of heuristics in pediatric pain management is important in knowledge translation.

Often, heuristics are used to quicken decision making or to deal with either very complex and plentiful information or gaps in one's knowledge. There are three basic types of heuristics *(147)*. The first is representativeness, basing a decision on how well a situation or person fits into a certain group (stereotyping). The second is availability, in which information that comes easily to mind influences a decision (flawed base rates). The last heuristic is anchoring and adjustment, in which an initial assessment, or an anchor, is made, which is then modified because of additional information (adjustment). However, the presence of the anchor affects the amount of adjustment caused by new information. The use of heuristics can be helpful as it facilitates making decisions quickly in an age when people are overwhelmed with information. However, heuristics may also lead to error resulting from flawed decision making, such as the overestimation of true rates of a condition.

We completed a supplementary analysis of the qualitative data in the research utilization studies to identify how nurses use heuristics in pediatric pain management decision making. We searched 137 field notes, 71 interview transcripts, and 10 focus group transcripts for pediatric pain-related decision-making events. We then analyzed those events. Using classic heuristic theory, we developed a coding scheme to categorize the events into the three traditional types of heuristics.

We found significant use of heuristic devices by nurses. Specifically, we found 16 cases of representativeness, 7 cases of availability, and 6 cases of anchoring and adjustment. In this sample, representativeness was the most widely used heuristic; the other two heuristic devices were used as well, but less frequently. The prevalence of decisions in which representativeness was used suggests that management of children's pain may be more generalized and less individualized. Where representativeness was analyzed, we noted that nurses (and much less frequently other health providers) using representativeness often assumed that certain surgical procedures were associated with certain levels of pain. This is especially problematic in pediatric pain management as infants and children are less able to communicate their pain or specifics about their pain to a health care professional. Infants and children also have more individualized methods of coping with pain than older people, who can rate their pain on standardized scales and communicate its severity. Representativeness can be beneficial in that health care professionals are more prepared for a certain condition, but it can be harmful in that health care professionals will be slower and more prone to error when treating a condition that was not expected. Ideally, all these heuristics have an appropriate place in the pain management decision-making process by adding speed and ability to deal with complex information; however, when providers are unaware of the potential erroneous conclusions to which their indiscriminate use may lead, the results may be erroneous pain interventions.

7. Solutions to the Knowledge Translation Problem

It is obvious that the relationship between knowledge and behavior is not linear or simple. Encouraging health care professionals to use research in their practice is compelling them to change their behavior—to change the way that they make decisions. Behavior change is complex, yet possible. Although there is a rich tradition in the cognitive sciences and among decision theorists of understanding the decision-making behaviors of health care professionals, it is relatively recent that we have seen any bridging of this work with that of the knowledge translation scientists. Therefore, much of the science of influencing decision making in combination with knowledge translation is in early development. We do find, however, some theoretical guidance in the literature to inform solutions to the knowledge translation challenge in pediatric pain management.

Building on the conclusions of Grimshaw and Eccles *(63)*, many of the interventions developed and tested to improve the effectiveness of research uptake have not been based on theory. The reality is that many times it is unclear from study reports why a particular intervention was chosen. Therefore, when proposing solutions to the knowledge translation problem in pediatric pain management, several points should be kept in mind. Future interventions to enhance the use of research in the management of children's pain must attend to the complex organizational contexts in which health care professionals work.

Solberg *(60)* suggested that designing organizational interventions that support the behavior change may be more appropriate than attempting to change individual behavior changes. What would this look like for pediatric pain management? It means designing systems that appreciate the complex, dynamic settings in which health care professionals make decisions and designing system changes with an appreciation for competing demands from multiple stakeholders. On a regular basis, pediatric health care professionals face multiple situations and people; these compete for their responses. A manifest challenge will be to develop interventions that enable them to give research more weight in their decisions.

Passive dissemination of pediatric pain research does not work. Therefore, interventions to improve the use of research in pediatric pain decision making may best focus on personal contact with pediatric pain practitioners, reminders, and interactive education meetings. Current wisdom suggests that interactions and linkages between researchers and decision makers are essential for optimum research uptake. Pain researchers and clinicians should then work much more closely and in a partnership model to address pain management challenges.

Our work within the Knowledge Utilization Studies program supports these types of interventions. It also strongly supports interventions designed to maximize and optimize the naturally occurring preference among health care professionals, especially nurses, for interactions as both a knowledge source and a problem-solving mechanism. Developing strategies to infuse research into these interactions and maximizing the involvement of colleagues who are respected and trusted is likely to be a successful strategy. How these interventions would "look" is unclear, but this approach holds considerable promise for increasing the uptake and use of research in pediatric pain management.

Other ongoing work in our program—work that has taken a more explicit "culture as variable" approach—originated in a 5-year funded program of research. Part of this program has focused on modeling research use across levels of decision making in organizations, as well as assessed the context dimension of the PARIHS (Promoting Action on Research Implementation in Health Services) *(120)* framework for research implementation. From these early findings, we have begun to appreciate that many of the interventions studied to date and much of the descriptive work, in nursing at least, has insufficiently accounted for both the work environments in which health providers are situated and the nature of the work of clinicians, or in our case, nurses. We believe that organizationally focused interventions in combination with interventions targeting individual levels of decision making—and assuming appropriately available *forms* of research evidence—will be necessary to develop meaningful intervention strategies.

8. Conclusions

Children continue to endure pain despite a well-established body of pediatric pain research evidence. There have been innumerable scientific advancements in the understanding, treatment, and management of pain in children, yet pediatric pain is still inadequately managed. In this chapter, we have argued that this is the result of the challenge in translating pediatric pain research into the clinical practices of health care providers. Although lack of knowledge remains a factor in many cases, this challenge is in fact a knowledge translation challenge, not a knowledge deficit one. In knowledge translation, research is considered along with numerous other sources of information and influences: personal preferences, professional group norms, the values of the organization or setting in which the decision is made, for example. Translating extant research into action is not easy because it demands that health care providers change their decision-making behaviors. Changing behaviors is complex, particularly if we consider the high-velocity, complex environments in which providers work and the influences that they face on a day-to-day basis.

In this chapter, we discussed challenges to the translation of pediatric pain research into practice, such as the values and beliefs that people hold about pain in children and the heuristics that providers use in making clinical decisions. Also, we offered potential approaches to close the gap between science and practice, in other words, to ensure that research is at the very least considered by providers when making pediatric pain management decisions. Interventions to increase the use of research in practice must attend to the complex and dynamic systems in which providers work. Providers do not work in isolation, and their decisions are subsequently influenced by their personal values, colleagues, patients, and the values held within their work environments, among other influences. This complex array of influences must be accounted for in strategies to increase the application of pediatric pain research in practice. The science of knowledge translation tells us that we cannot continue with present dissemination behaviors and hope that providers will simply use what we publish in scientific journals. Passive dissemination is not enough; clearly, more innovative strategies to facilitate the infusion of research into decision-making processes and provider behaviors are required.

References

1. Hamilton SM, Letourneau S, Pekeles E, Voaklander D, Johnston DWCJ. The impact of regionalization on a surgery program in the Canadian health care system. Arch Surg 1997;132:605–611.
2. Howard MO, McMillen CJ, Pollio DE. Teaching evidence-based practice: toward a new paradigm for social work education. Res Soc Work Pract 2003;13:234–260.
3. Tesler MD, Wilkie DJ, Holzemer WL, Savedra MC. Postoperative analgesics for children and adolescents: prescription and administration. J Pain Symptom Manage 1994;9:85–95.
4. Sung N. Central challenges facing the national clinical research enterprise. JAMA 2003;289:1278–1287.
5. Grol R. Successes and failures in the implementation of evidence-based guidelines for clinical practice. Med Care 2001;39(8, supplement 2):II-46–II-54.
6. Schuster M, McGlynn E, Brook R. How good is the quality of health care in the United States? Milbank Q 1998;76:517–563.
7. Anand K. Clinical importance of pain and stress in preterm neonates. Biol Neonate 1998;73:1–9.
8. Anand K. Pain, plasticity and premature birth: a prescription for permanent suffering? Nat Med 2000;6:971–973.
9. Fitzgerald M. Pain in infancy: some unanswered questions. Pain Rev 1995;2:77–91.
10. Anand K, Brown M, Bloom S, Aynsley-Green A. Studies on the hormonal regulation of fuel metabolism in the human newborn infant undergoing anaesthesia and surgery. Horm Res 1985;22:115–128.
11. Anand K, Hickey P. Pain and its effect in the human neonate and fetus. N Engl J Med 1987;317:1321–1329.
12. Whaley L, Wong D. Whaley and Wong's Nursing Care of Infants and Children. St. Louis, MO: Mosby Year Book; 1999.
13. Warnock F, Lander J. Pain progression, intensity and outcomes following tonsillectomy. Pain 1998;75:37–45.
14. Lander J. Fallacies and phobias about addiction and pain. Br J Addict 1990;85:803–809.
15. The Jason Program. Joint Scientific Meeting of the American Pain Society and Canadian Pain Society [Web page]. 2004. Available at: www.jasonprogram.org/pediatric_pain.htm. Accessed September 7, 2004.

16. Landry R, Amara N, Lamari M. Utilization of social science research knowledge in Canada. Res Policy 2001;30:333–349.
17. Glaser EM, Abelson HH, Garrison KN. Putting Knowledge to Use. San Francisco: Jossey-Bass; 1983.
18. Mosteller F. Innovation and evaluation. Science 1981;211:881–886.
19. Rogers E. Diffusion of Innovations. 4th ed. New York: Free Press; 1995.
20. Stastny P, Ichinose T, Thayer S, Olson R, Keens T. Infant sleep positioning by nursery staff and mothers in newborn hospital nurseries. Nurs Res 2004;53:122–129.
21. Larsen JK. Knowledge utilization. What is it? Knowledge: Creation, Diffusion, Utilization 1980;1:421–442.
22. Evidence-Based Medicine Working Group. Evidence-based medicine. A new approach to teaching the practice of medicine. JAMA 1992;268:2420–2425.
23. Gray M. Scientific truths: weighing the evidence. J Wound Ostomy Continence Nurs 1995;22:203–205.
24. National Forum on Health. Canada Health Action: Building on the Legacy. Ottawa: National Forum on Health; 1997.
25. Ketefian S. Application of selected nursing research findings into nursing practice. Nurs Res 1975;24:89–92.
26. Shore HL. Adopters and laggards. Can Nurse 1972;68:36–39.
27. Horsley JA, Crane J, Bingle JD. Research utilization as an organizational process. J Nurs Adm 1978;8:4–6.
28. Horsley JA, Crane J, Crabtree MK, Wood DJ. Using Research to Improve Nursing Practice: a Guide. San Fransisco: Grune and Stratton; 1983.
29. Estabrooks CA, Scott-Findlay S, Winther C. Knowledge utilization in nursing and the allied health sciences. In: Champagne F, Lemieux-Charles L, eds. Multidisciplinary Perspectives on Evidence-Based Decision-Making in Health Care. Toronto: University of Toronto; 2004:242–295.
30. Canadian Institutes of Health Research. Knowledge translation (KT) [Web page]. Available at: http://www.cihr-irsc.gc.ca/e/8505.html. Accessed November 23, 2004.
31. Smith R. Doctors are not scientists. BMJ 2004;328:doi:10.1136–bmj.328.7454.0-4.
32. Greenhalgh T, Robert G, Bate P. How to Spread Good Ideas: a Systematic Review of the Literature on Diffusion, Dissemination and Sustainability of Innovations in Health Service Delivery and Organisation. Report for the National Coordinating Centre for NHS Service Delivery and Organisation. Leeds, UK: National Coordinating Centre for NHS Service Delivery and Organisation, 2004.
33. Rogers EM. Lessons for guidelines from the diffusion of innovations. Jt Comm J Qual Improv 1995;21:324–328.
34. Rice RE, Rogers EM. Reinvention in the innovation process. Knowledge: Creation, Diffusion, Utilization 1980;1:499–514.
35. Lemieux-Charles L, Barnsley J. An innovation diffusion perspective on knowledge and evidence in health care. In: Lemieux-Charles L, Champagne F, eds. Using Knowledge and Evidence in Health Care: Multidisciplinary Perspectives. Toronto: University of Toronto Press; 2004:115–138.
36. Estabrooks CA. Translating research into practice: implications for organizations and administrators. Can J Nurs Res 2003;35:53–68.

37. Jacoby J. Personality and innovation proneness. J Mark Res 1971;8:244–247.
38. Mohr L. Determinants of innovation in organizations. Am Polit Sci Rev 1969;63: 111–126.
39. Kimberly J. Organizational and contextual influences on the diffusion of technological innovation. In: Pennings JM, Buitendam A, eds. New Technology as Organizational Innovation. Cambridge, UK: Ballinger; 1987:237–259.
40. Rogers EM. Diffusion of Innovations. 3rd ed. New York: Free Press; 1983.
41. Warner K. The need for some innovative concepts of innovation: an examination of research on the diffusion of innovations. Policy Sci 1974;5:433–451.
42. Scott S, Bruce R. Determinants of innovative behaviour: a path model of individual innovation in the workplace. Acad Manage J 1994;37:580–607.
43. Morrow-Bradley C, Elliott R. Utilization of psychotherapy research by practicing psychotherapists. Am Psychol 1986;41:188–197.
44. Cohen L, Sargent M, Sechrest L. Use of psychotherapy research by professional psychologist. Am Psychol 1986;4:198–206.
45. Estabrooks CA, Floyd JA, Scott-Findlay S, O'Leary KA, Gushta M. Individual determinants of research utilization: a systematic review. J Adv Nurs 2003;43:506–520.
46. Grimshaw JM, Russell IT. Effect of clinical guidelines on medical practice: a systematic review of rigorous evaluations. Lancet 1993;342:1317–1321.
47. Woolf SH, Grol R, Hutchinson A, Eccles M, Grimshaw JW. Potential benefits, limitations, and harms of clinical guidelines. BMJ 1999;318:527–530.
48. Haynes R. Of studies, summaries, synopses and systems: the "4S" evolution of services for finding current best evidence. Evid Based Ment Health 2001; 4:37–39.
49. Hunt DL, Haynes RB, Hanna SE, Smith K. Effects of computer-based clinical decision support systems on physician performance and patient outcomes. A systematic review. JAMA 1998;280:1339–1346.
50. Wyatt J, Paterson-Brown S, Johanson R, Altman D, Bradburn M, Fisk N. Randomized trial of educational visits to enhance use of systematic reviews in 25 obstetric units. BMJ 1998;317:1041–1046.
51. Davies D, Thomson O'Brien M, Freemantle N, Wolf F, Mazmanian P, Taylor-Vaisey A. Impact of formal continuing medical education: do conferences, workshops, rounds and other traditional continuing education activities change physician behaviour or healthcare outcomes? JAMA 1999;282:867–874.
52. Oxman AD, Thomson MA, Davis DA, Haynes RB. No magic bullets: a systematic review of 102 trials of interventions to help health care professionals deliver services more effectively or efficiently. Can Med Assoc J 1995;153:1423–1431.
53. Bero L, Grilli R, Grimshaw JM, Harvey E, Oxman A, Thomson MA. Closing the gap between research and practice: an overview of systematic reviews of interventions to promote implementation of research findings. BMJ 1998;317:465–468.
54. Freemantle N, Harvey EL, Wolf F, Grimshaw JM, Grilli R, Bero LA. Printed educational materials: effects on professional practice and health care outcomes. Cochrane Database Syst Rev 1997;2.

55. Thomson O'Brien MA, Oxman AD, Haynes RB, Davis DA, Freemantle N, Harvey EL. Local opinion leaders: effects on professional practice and health care outcomes. Cochrane Database Syst Rev 1999;1.

56. Effective Health Care. Getting evidence into practice. Effective Health Care Bull 1999;5:1–16.

57. Grol R, Grimshaw J. Evidence-based implementation of evidence-based medicine. Jt Comm J Qual Improv 1999;25:503–513.

58. Thomson O'Brien MA, Oxman AD, Davis DA, Haynes RB, Freemantle N, Harvey EL. Audit feedback vs alternative strategies: effects on professional practice and health care outcomes. Cochrane Library 2003;1.

59. Grimshaw JM, Shirran L, Thomas R, et al. Changing provider behavior: an overview of systematic reviews of interventions. Med Care 2001;39(8, suppl 2):II-2–II-45.

60. Solberg L. Guideline implementation: what the literature doesn't tell us. Jt Comm J Qual Improv 2000;26:525–537.

61. Gross P, Greenfield S, Cretin S, et al. Optimal methods for guideline implementation: conclusion from Leeds Castle meeting. Med Care 2001;39(8, suppl 2): II-85–II92.

62. Grimshaw JM, Thomas RE, MacIennan G, et al. Effectiveness and efficiency of guideline dissemination and implementation strategies. Health Technol Assess 2004;8:1–72.

63. Grimshaw J, Eccles M. Is evidence-based implementation of evidence-based care possible? Med J Aust 2004;180:S50, S51.

64. Grol R. Personal paper: beliefs and evidence in changing clinical practice. BMJ 1997;315:418–421.

65. Medical Research Council. A framework for development and evaluation of RCTs for complex interventions to improve health [Web page]. 2000. Available at: www.mrc.ac.uk/pdf-mrc_cpr.pdf. Accessed October 1, 2004.

66. Perri M. The maintenance of treatment effects in the long-term management of obesity. Clin Psychol Sci Pract 1998;5:526–543.

67. United States National Cancer Institute. Theory at a glance: a guide for health promotion practice [Web page]. 2003. Available at: http://www.cancer.gov/about-nci/oc/theory-at-a-glance. Accessed September 23, 2004.

68. Field M, Lohr K. Clinical Practice Guidelines: Directions of a New Program. Washington, DC: Institute of Medicine; 1990.

69. Fowler FJ Jr, Gallagher PM, Stringfellow VL, Zaslavsky AM, Thompson JW, Cleary PD. Using telephone interviews to reduce nonresponse bias to mail surveys of health plan members. Med Care 2002;40:190–200.

70. Grimshaw J, Eccles M, Russell I. Developing clinically valid practice guidelines. J Eval Clin Pract 1995;1:37–48.

71. Grimshaw J, Hutchinson A. Clinical practice guidelines do they enhance value for money in healthcare? Br Med Bull 1995;51:927–940.

72. Jousimaa J, Makeka M, Kunnamo I, MacLennan G, Grimshaw J. Primary care guidelines on consultation practices: the effectiveness of computerized vs paper-based versions. Int J Technol Assess Health Care 2002;18:586–596.

73. Lomas J. Connecting research and policy. Isuma 2000;1:140–144.
74. McGrath P. Pain in Children: Nature, Assessment and Treatment. New York: Guilford; 1990.
75. World Health Organization. Myths and misconceptions about pain control in children [Web page]. Available at: http://www.whocancerpain.wisc.edu/eng/16_3-4/mths.html. Accessed October 8, 2004.
76. Ferlie E, Shortell S. Improving the quality of health care in the United Kingdom and the United States: a framework for change. Milbank Q 2001;72:281–315.
77. Damanpour F. Organizational complexity and innovation: developing and testing multiple contingency models. Manage Sci 1996;42:693–716.
78. Meyer A, Goes J. Organizational assimilation of innovations: a multilevel contextual analysis. Acad Manage Rev 1988;31:897–923.
79. Orlandi M. The diffusion and adoption of worksite health promotion innovations: an analysis of barriers. Prev Med 1986;15:522–536.
80. Damanpour F. The adoption of technological, administrative, and ancillary innovations: impact of organizational factors. J Manage 1987;13:675–688.
81. Damanpour F. Organizational innovation: a meta-analysis of effects of determinants and moderators. Acad Manage J 1991;34:555–590.
82. Kimberly J. Managerial innovation. In: Nystrom PSW, ed. Handbook of Organizational Design. Vol. 1. Oxford, UK: Oxford University Press; 1981:84–104.
83. Kimberly J, Evanisko M. Organizational innovation: the influence of individual, organizational, and contextual factors on hospital adoption of technological and administrative innovations. Acad Manage J 1981;24:689–713.
84. Moch M, Morse E. Size, centralization and organizational adoption of innovations. Am Sociol Rev 1977;42:716–725.
85. Germain R. The role of context and structure in radical and incremental logistics innovation adoption. J Bus Res 1996;35:117–127.
86. Zmud R. An examination of "push-pull" theory applied to process innovation in knowledge work. Manage Sci 1984;30:727–738.
87. Varcoe C, Hilton A. Factors affecting acute-care nurses' use of research findings. Can J Nurs Res 1995;27:51–71.
88. Brett JLL. Use of nursing practice research findings. Nurs Res 1987;36:344–349.
89. Brett JLL. Organizational integrative mechanisms and adoption of innovations by nurses. Nurs Res 1989;38:105–110.
90. Chakrabarti A. The role of champion in product innovation. Calif Manage Rev 1974;17:58–62.
91. Howell J, Higgins C. Champions of change: identifying understanding, and supporting champions of technological innovations. Organ Dyn 1990;19:40–55.
92. Markham S, Green S, Basu R. Champions and antagonists: relationships with R&D project characteristics and management. J Eng Technol Manage 1991;8:217–242.
93. Schon D. Champions for radical new inventions. Harv Bus Rev 1963;March–April:77–86.
94. Thompson G, Degner L, Estabrooks C. Ambiguous roles: a literature review clarifying concepts used in knowledge utilization and dissemination. J Adv Nurs 2004.

95. Downs G, Mohr L. Conceptual issues in the study of innovation. Adm Sci Q 1976;21:700–714.

96. Fennell M. Synergy, influence, and information in the adoption of administrative innovations. Acad Manage J 1984;27:113–129.

97. Zaltman G, Duncan R, Holbek J. Innovations and Organizations. Toronto: Wiley; 1973.

98. Funk SG, Champagne MT, Wiese RA, Tornquist EM. BARRIERS: The barriers to research utilization scale. Appl Nurs Res 1991;4:39–45.

99. Humphris D, Littlejohns P, Victor C, O'Halloran P, Peacock J. Implementing evidence-based practice: factors that influence the use of research evidence by occupational therapists. Br J Occup Ther 2000;63:516–522.

100. Pettengill MM, Gillies DA, Clark CC. Factors encouraging and discouraging the use of nursing research findings. Image J Nurs Sch 1994;26:143–147.

101. Rodgers S. An exploratory study of research utilization by nurses in general medical and surgical wards. J Adv Nurs 1994;20:904–911.

102. Richens Y. Are midwives using research evidence in practice? Br J Midwifery 2001;9:237–242.

103. Rizzuto C, Bostrom J, Newton Suter W, Chenitz WC. Predictors of nurses' involvement in research activities. West J Nurs Res 1994;16:193–204.

104. Rodgers SE. The extent of nursing research utilization in general medical and surgical wards. J Adv Nurs 2000;32:182–193.

105. Walczak JR, McGuire DB, Haisfield ME, Beezley A. A survey of research-related activities and perceived barriers to research utilization among professional oncology nurses. Oncol Nurs Forum 1994;21:710–715.

106. Champion VL, Leach A. Variables related to research utilization in nursing: an empirical investigation. J Adv Nurs 1989;14:705–710.

107. Clifford C, Murray S. Pre- and post-test evaluation of a project to facilitate research development in practice in a hospital setting. J Adv Nurs 2001;36:685–695.

108. Royle J, Blythe J, Ciliska D, Ing D. The organizational environment and evidence-based nursing. Can J Nurs Leadersh 2000;13:31–37.

109. Royle JA, Blythe J, DiCenso A, Boblin-Cummings S, Deber R, Hayward R. Evaluation of a system for providing information resources to nurses. Health Informatics J 2000;5:100–109.

110. Hefferin EA, Horsley JA, Ventura MR. Promoting research-based nursing: the nurse administrator's role. J Nurs Adm 1982;May:34–41.

111. Lacey EA. Facilitating research-based practice by educational intervention. Nurse Educ Today 1996;16:296–301.

112. Aiken LH, Clarke SP, Sloane DM, Sochalski JA. An international perspective on hospital nurses' work environments: the case for reform. Policy Polit Nurs Pract 2001;2:255–263.

113. Aiken LH, Clarke SP, Sloane DM, et al. Nurses' reports of hospital quality of care and working conditions in five countries. Health Aff 2001;20:43–53.

114. Aiken LH, Patrician PA. Measuring organizational traits in hospitals: the revised nursing work index. 2000;49:146–153.

115. Hatcher S, Tranmer J. A survey of variables related to research utilization in nursing practice in the acute care setting. Can J Nurs Adm 1997;Sept–Oct:31–53.

116. Lacey EA. Research utilization in nursing practice—a pilot study. J Adv Nurs 1994;19:987–995.

117. Alcock D, Carroll G, Goodman M. Staff nurses' perceptions of factors influencing their role in research. Can J Nurs Res 1990;22:7–18.

118. Bostrom J, Suter WN. Research utilization: making the link to practice. J Nurses Staff Dev 1993;9:28–34.

119. Nelson D. Research into research practice. Accid Emerg Nurs 1995;3:184–189.

120. Coyle LA, Sokop AG. Innovation adoption behavior among nurses. Nurs Res 1990;39:176–180.

121. Kitson A, Harvey G, McCormack B. Enabling the implementation of evidence based practice: a conceptual framework. Qual Health Care 1998;7:149–158.

122. McCormack B, Kitson A, Harvey G, Rycroft-Malone J, Titchen A, Seers K. Getting evidence into practice: the meaning of "context." J Adv Nurs 2002;38: 94–104.

123. Rycroft-Malone J, Kitson A, Harvey G, et al. Ingredients for change: revisiting a conceptual framework. Qual Saf Health Care 2002;11:174–180.

124. Feldman SP. Management in context: an essay on the relevance of culture to the understanding of organizational change. J Manage Stud 1986;23:587–607.

125. Fiol M, Hatch MJ, Golden-Biddle K. Relationships between culture and identity. In: Whetten D, ed. Identity in Organizations: Developing Theory Through Conversations. Thousand Oaks, CA: Sage; 1998, pp. 56–59.

126. Golden KA. The individual and organizational culture: strategies for action in highly ordered contexts. J Manage Stud 1992;29:1–22.

127. Hatch M. The dynamics of organizational culture. Acad Manage Rev 1993;18: 657–693.

128. Hatch MJ. Organization Theory: Modern, Symbolic and Postmodern Perspectives. New York: Oxford University Press; 1997.

129. Meyerson D, Martin J. Cultural change: an integration of three different views. J Manage Stud 1987;24:623–647.

130. Smircich L. Concepts of culture and organizational analysis. Adm Sci Q 1983;28: 339–358.

131. Schein EH. Organizational Culture and Leadership. 2nd ed. San Francisco: Jossey-Bass; 1992.

132. Hatch, M. Dynamics in organizational culture [Web page]. 2003. Available at: http://www.commerce.virginia.edu/faculty_research/Research/Papers/Hatch_Dy namics_Organizational_Culture.pdf. Accessed August 3, 2004.

133. Aiken LH, Clarke SP, Sloane DM, Sochalski J, Silber JH. Hospital nurse staffing and patient mortality, nurse burnout, and job dissatisfaction. JAMA 2002;288:1987–1993.

134. Needleman J, Buerhaus P, Mattke S, Stewart M, Zelevinsky K. Nurse-staffing levels and the quality of care in hospitals. N Engl J Med 2002;346:1715–1722.

135. Lave J, Wenger E. Situated Learning: Legitimate Peripheral Participation. Cambridge, UK: Cambridge University Press; 1991.

136. Wenger E. Communities of Practice: Learning, Meaning, and Identity. Cambridge, UK: Cambridge University Press; 1998.

137. Estabrooks CA, Scott-Findlay S, Rutukumwa W, Duan Q, O'Leary K, Rozanova J. The Determinants of Research Utilization Studies. KUSP Technical Report. Edmonton, Alberta, Canada: University of Alberta; 2004.

138. Eisenhardt K. Speed and strategic choice: how managers accelerate decision making. Calif Manage Rev 1990;Spring:39–54.

139. Eisenhardt K. Speed and strategic choice: accelerating decision-making. Planning Rev 1992;20:30–32.

140. Baessler CA, Blumbert M, Cunningham JS, et al. Medical-surgical nurses' utilization of research methods and products. Medsurg Nursing 1994;3:113–117, 120–121, 141.

141. Estabrooks CA, Chong H, Brigidear K, Profetto-McGrath J. Profiling Canadian nurses' preferred knowledge sources for clinical practice. Can J Nurs Res 2005; 37:118–140.

142. Estabrooks CA. Will evidence-based nursing practice make practice perfect? Can J Nurs Res 1998;30:15–36.

143. Estabrooks C, Rutakumwa W, O'Leary K, et al. Sources of practice knowledge among nurses. Qual Health Res 2005;15:470–476.

144. Estabrooks C, Scott-Findlay S, Milner M, et al. Factors that influence nurses' choice of knowledge sources. Can J Nurs Res, under review.

145. Chapman G, Sonnenberg F. Decision making in healthcare: theory, psychology and applications. Cambridge, UK: Cambridge University Press; 2000.

146. Patel VL, Kaufman DR, Arocha JF. Emerging paradigms of cognition in medical decision-making. J Biomed Inform 2002;35:52–75.

147. Tversky A, Kahneman D. Judgment Under Certainty: Heuristics and Biases. New York: Cambridge University Press; 1974.

Index